P9-DVF-785

R. Tadeusiewicz, M. R. Ogiela

Medical Image Understanding Technology

Springer

Berlin
Heidelberg
New York
Hong Kong
London
Milano
Paris
Tokyo

Studies in Fuzziness and Soft Computing, Volume 156

Editor-in-chief
Prof. Janusz Kacprzyk
Systems Research Institute
Polish Academy of Sciences
ul. Newelska 6
01-447 Warsaw
Poland
E-mail: kacprzyk@ibspan.waw.pl

Further volumes of this series
can be found on our homepage:
springeronline.com

Vol. 140. A. Abraham, L.C. Jain,
B.J. van der Zwaag (Eds.)
Innovations in Intelligent Systems, 2004
ISBN 3-540-20265-X

Vol. 141. G.C. Onwubolu, B.V. Babu
New Optimzation Techniques in Engineering, 2004
ISBN 3-540-20167-X

Vol. 142. M. Nikravesh, L.A. Zadeh,
V. Korotkikh (Eds.)
Fuzzy Partial Differential Equations and Relational Equations, 2004
ISBN 3-540-20322-2

Vol. 143. L. Rutkowski
New Soft Computing Techniques for System Modelling, Pattern Classification and Image Processing, 2004
ISBN 3-540-20584-5

Vol. 144. Z. Sun, G.R. Finnie
Intelligent Techniques in E-Commerce, 2004
ISBN 3-540-20518-7

Vol. 145. J. Gil-Aluja
Fuzzy Sets in the Management of Uncertainty, 2004
ISBN 3-540-20341-9

Vol. 146. J.A. Gámez, S. Moral, A. Salmerón (Eds.)
Advances in Bayesian Networks, 2004
ISBN 3-540-20876-3

Vol. 147. K. Watanabe, M.M.A. Hashem
New Algorithms and their Applications to Evolutionary Robots, 2004
ISBN 3-540-20901-8

Vol. 148. C. Martin-Vide, V. Mitrana,
G. Păun (Eds.)
Formal Languages and Applications, 2004
ISBN 3-540-20907-7

Vol. 149. J.J. Buckley
Fuzzy Statistics, 2004
ISBN 3-540-21084-9

Vol. 150. L. Bull (Ed.)
Applications of Learning Classifier Systems, 2004
ISBN 3-540-21109-8

Vol. 151. T. Kowalczyk, E. Pleszczyńska,
F. Ruland (Eds.)
Grade Models and Methods for Data Analysis, 2004
ISBN 3-540-21120-9

Vol. 152. J. Rajapakse, L. Wang (Eds.)
Neural Information Processing: Research and Development, 2004
ISBN 3-540-21123-3

Vol. 153. J. Fulcher, L.C. Jain (Eds.)
Applied Intelligent Systems, 2004
ISBN 3-540-21153-5

Vol. 154. B. Liu
Uncertainty Theory, 2004
ISBN 3-540-21333-3

Vol. 155. G. Resconi, J.L. Jain
Intelligent Agents, 2004
ISBN 3-540-22003-8

Ryszard Tadeusiewicz
Marek R. Ogiela

Medical Image Understanding Technology

Artificial Intelligence and Soft-Computing for Image Understanding

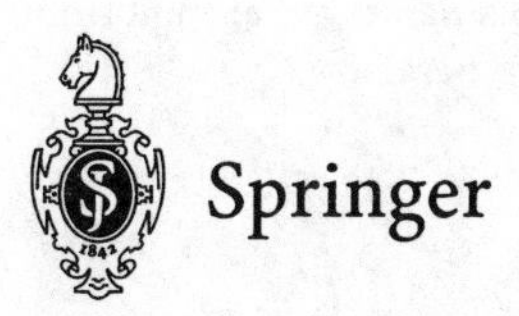

Springer

Professor Ryszard Tadeusiewicz
Professor Marek R. Ogiela
Department of Bio Cybernetics
AGH University of Science & Technology
30-059 Kraków
Poland
E-mail: mogiela@agh.edu.pl

ISSN 1434-9922
ISBN 3-540-21985-4 Springer-Verlag Berlin Heidelberg New York

Library of Congress Control Number: 2004105114

Springer-Verlag is a part of Springer Science+Business Media
springeronline.com

Printed in Germany

Typesetting: camera-ready by authors
Cover design: E. Kirchner, Springer-Verlag, Heidelberg
Printed on acid free paper 62/3020/M - 5 4 3 2 1 0

Contents

Introduction

This book proposes a new approach to the processing and analysis of medical images. We introduce the term (and methodology) medical data understanding, as a new step in the way of starting from image processing, and followed by analysis and classification (recognition). The general view of the situation of new technology under consideration in the context of the more well known techniques of image processing, analysis, segmentation and classification is shown below.

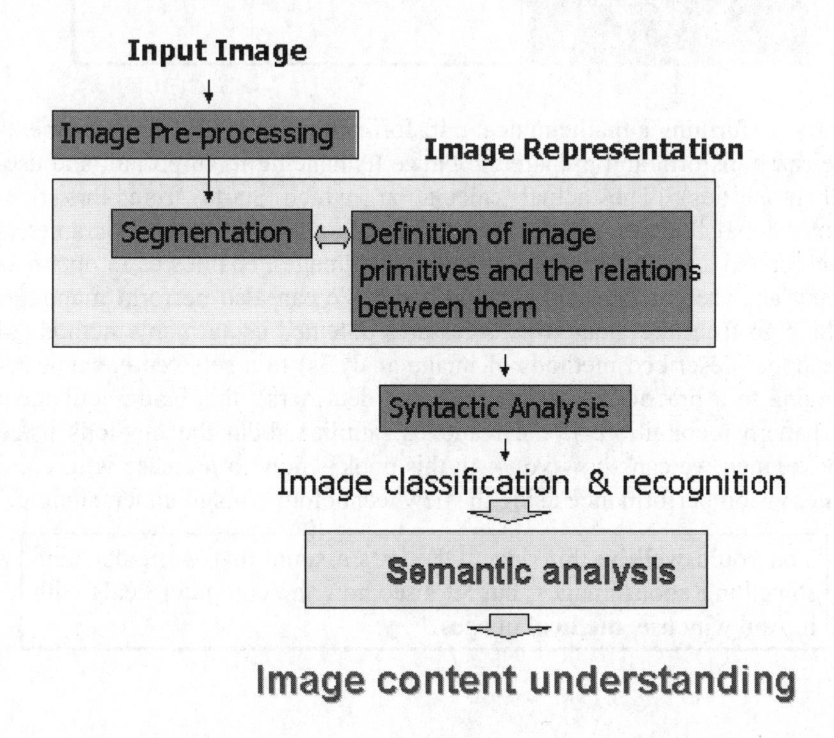

We assume that the reader is a little familiar with the general ideas that computer vision is a new branch of computer science based on the fact that every image can be presented as a two-dimensional function (see below).

All image processing techniques exist because each image can be presented as a two-dimensional function

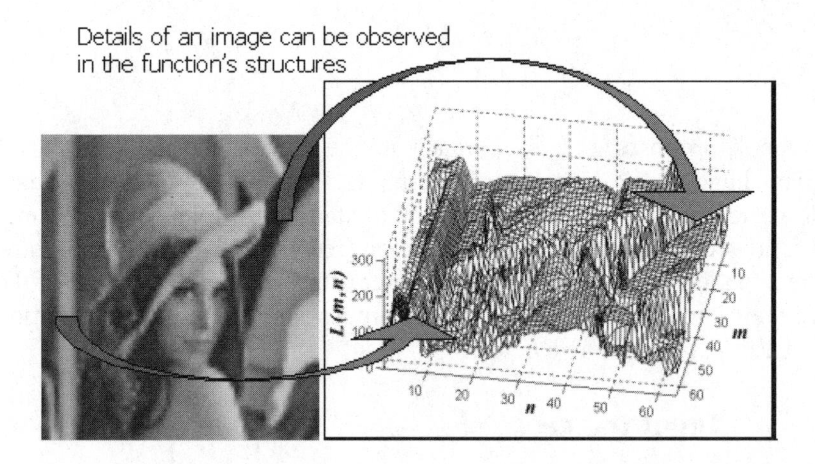

By performing a mathematical transformation of the function's elements we can transform and prepare the image (enhancing its important and useful properties). The actual calculation, which starts from this two-dimensional function but leads to values of some pre-selected parameters (interpreted as features of the object on the image), enables us to obtain as many analyses of the image as we need. We can also perform mappings which go from the image (or its features obtained using many methods of the upper described methods of image analysis) to a selected element belonging to a predefined set of symbols (identifiers); this being equivalent to pattern recognition. If the reader is familiar about the methods listed above, then we can show you – in this book – how to increase your computer vision performance using the new technology: image understanding.

You could well be thinking: 'OK, let's assume that we understand something about images, but let's see how the computer deals with it. And why use **medical** images?'

Lets compare two examples of ERCP images of the pancreatic duct with pancreatitis (permanent inflammation)

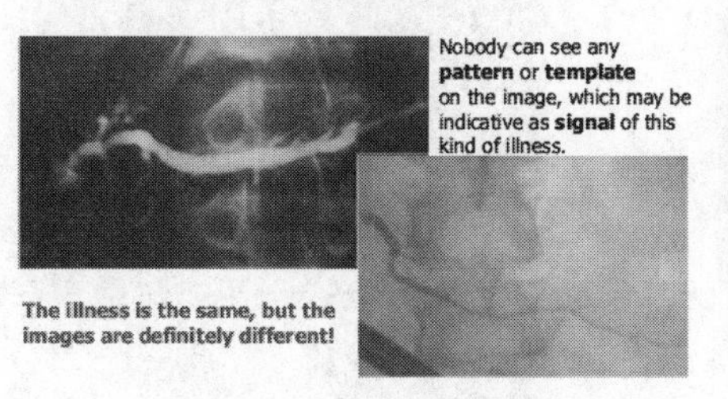

We find the same situation when analyzing ERCP images showing pancreatic cancer

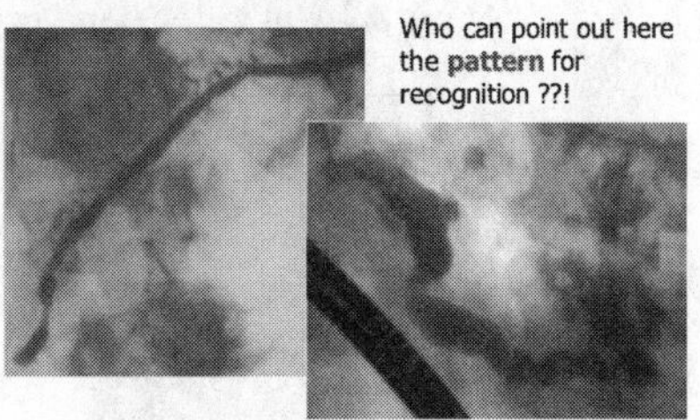

A more detailed analysis of this problem will be carried out inside the book, but your acceptance of the general idea of understanding medical images is very important for us, and we would like to show you some examples of medical images, which should be first **understood** rather than purely recognised.

Another typical example: cardiological imaging (coronarography) with evident symptoms of serious cardiac illnesses

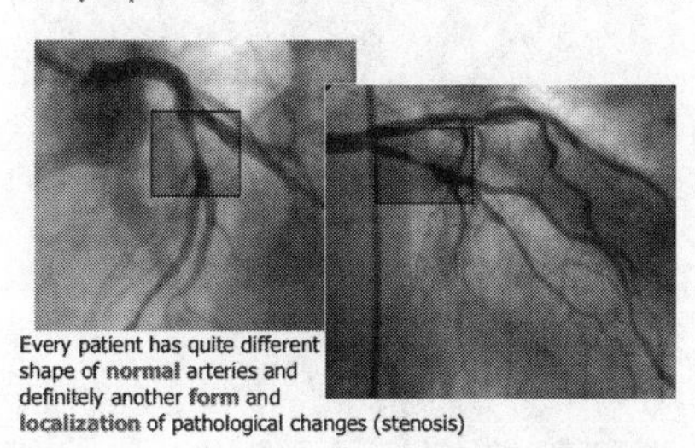

Similar problems one can find during analysis of X-ray images of ureters and kidney pelvis imaging (with pathological narrowing and other possible deformations)

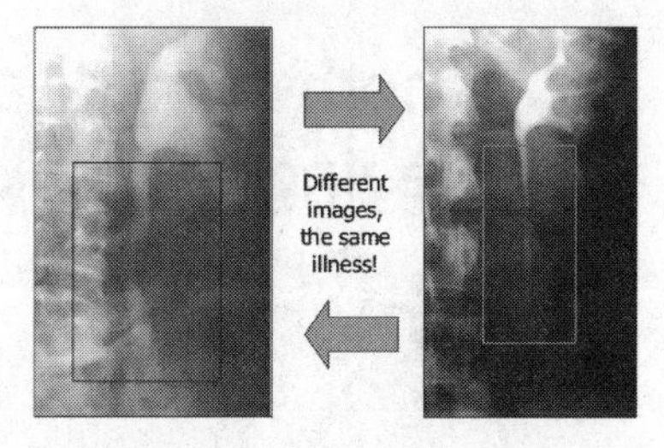

As you can see on the presented images – simple analysis and pattern recognition is completely insufficient for many medical applications, and we need to discover a new methodology that will be more efficient in helping physicians and for the better preservation of our common health.

In the following chapters of this book we try to show, that image understanding technology, as a next step after pattern recognition is useful, (sometimes even necessary), possible and also effective. This will be carried out using three types of medical images:

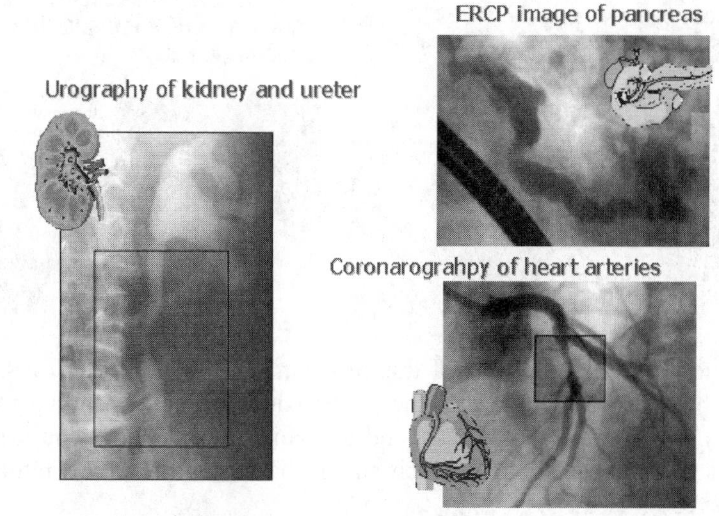

But in fact the methods under consideration can be used also for many other kinds of medical images.

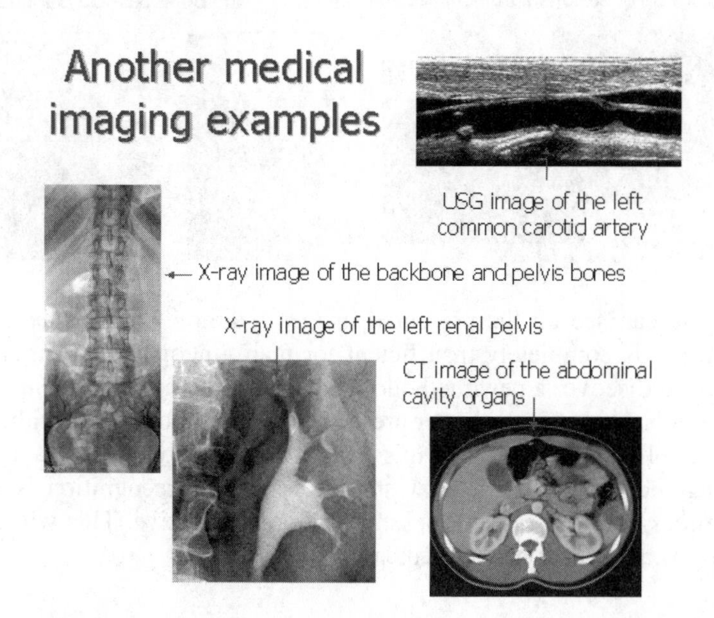

Of particular interest is the possibility of extending the methods described in this book for the understanding of images of the brain and (in other sense) for histological and histopathological images.

Brain Images

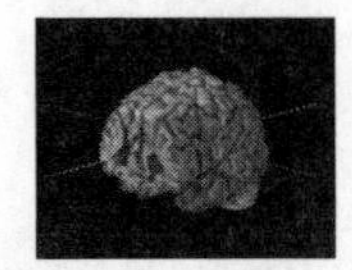

Images of Microscopic Structure and Tissue

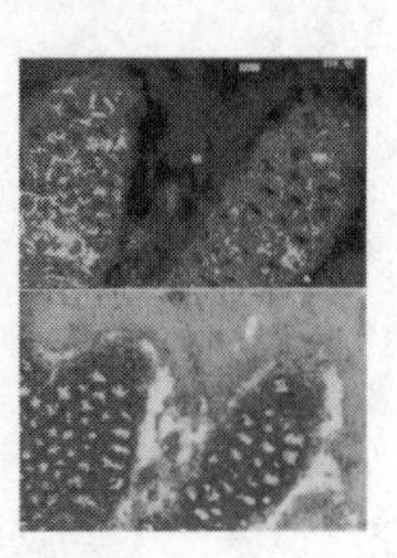

MRI image of cerebral hemispheres

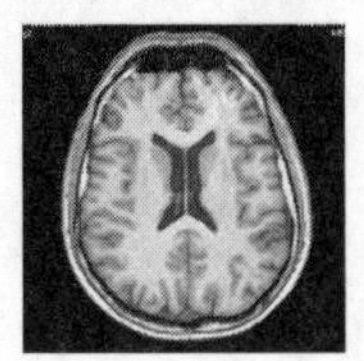

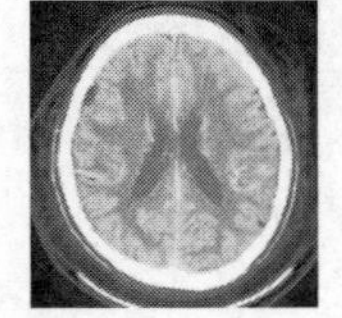

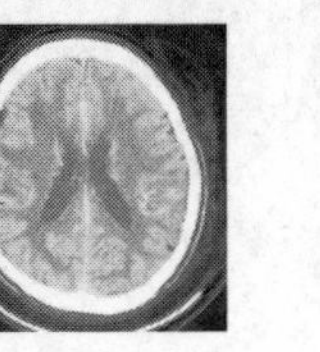

CT image of cerebral hemispheres

The content of the book is scheduled according to the goals described in previous paragraphs. In Chapter 1 we seek to explain, why and when this new technology can used. In Chapter 2 we then try to provide a general (intuitive) outline of the new concept of 'image understanding'. In Chapter 3 we give a detailed description of the so called syntactic methods for pattern recognition, which are the most important element of the proposed methodology. The Chapters that follow (4 and 5) are devoted to the description of selected examples and the use of the proposed methodology in solving of selected problems. The final chapter of this book is dedicated to the analysis of property strengths and weaknesses properties of the methods under consideration. A long and comprehensive bibliography provides references to the publications of other authors from which the more interested reader can find detailed information that is not listed in this book owing to its scope.

1. What is Image Understanding Technology and why do we need it?

1.1 Methods of Medical Image Acquisition

Medical procedures which involve the use of various images constitute a particularly interesting and important field of informatics, especially as contemporary medical diagnosis is to a large extent based on images. *Medical Imaging Technology* has now become one of the major sources of information for therapy and also for research in medicine, biology and in other related fields. This information covers the morphology of examined organs and their function (though in a limited degree), which affords us the means to infer whether their functioning is correct and whether the structures are pathological. This allows well-founded conclusions to be drawn or helps in modern diagnostic reasoning processes.

Advanced Medical Imaging Techniques provide us with various physical processes so that the researcher is easily and conveniently supplied with the required images. Medical imaging still uses classical X-ray techniques based on the fact that the amount of X-ray energy absorbed by particular tissues differs. The required imaging in this case is obtained either by using simple principles of geometric optics (whereby the source of X-radiation is treated as a particle and the shadows of examined organs are registered on the film or with the use of CCD detectors). Thus we can easily obtain images of the examined body parts (for example, of a broken leg – Fig. 1.1), organs (a mammogram – Fig. 1.2. or a RTG stomach image – Fig. 1.3) or a selected fragment of the examined organ, such as a vessel or duct filled with a contrast (Endoscopy Retrograde Cholagio-Pancretaography ERCP – Fig. 1.4, Urography – Fig. 1.5 or Coronarography – Fig.1.6).

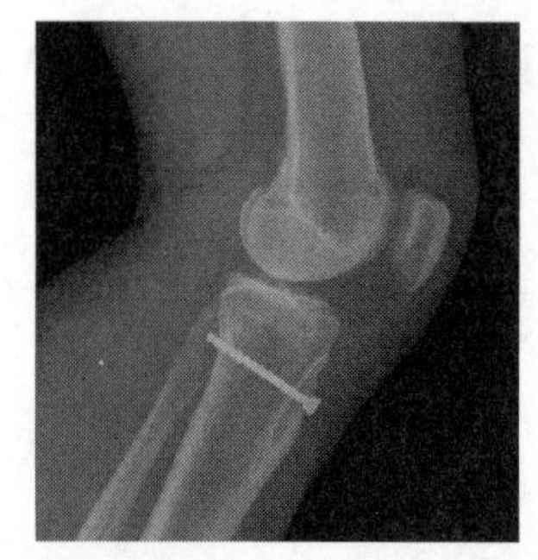

Fig. 1.1. Image of broken leg

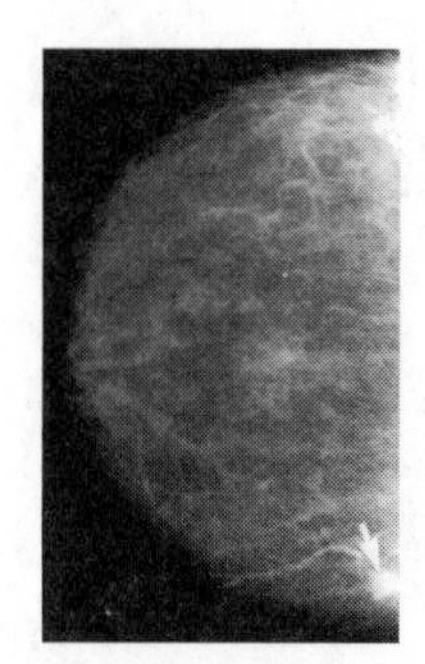

Fig. 1.2. Mammogram image

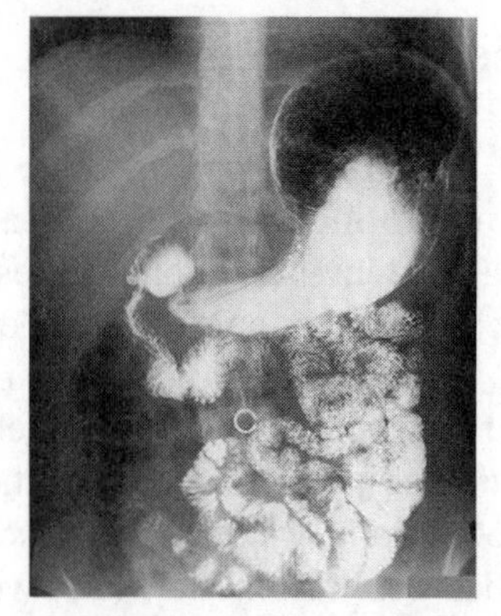

Fig. 1.3. RTG stomach image

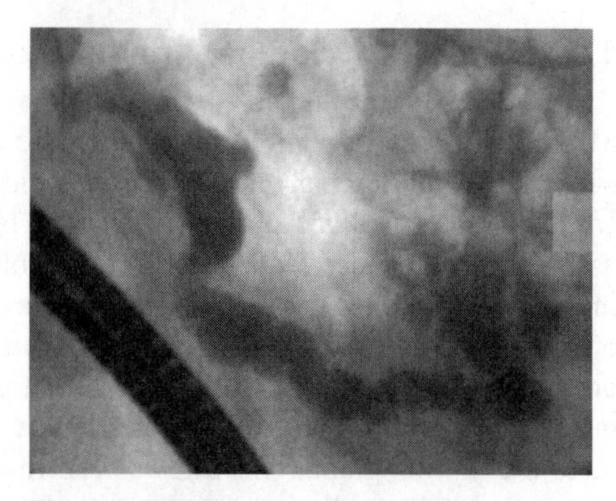

Fig. 1.4. ERCP image of pancreatic duct

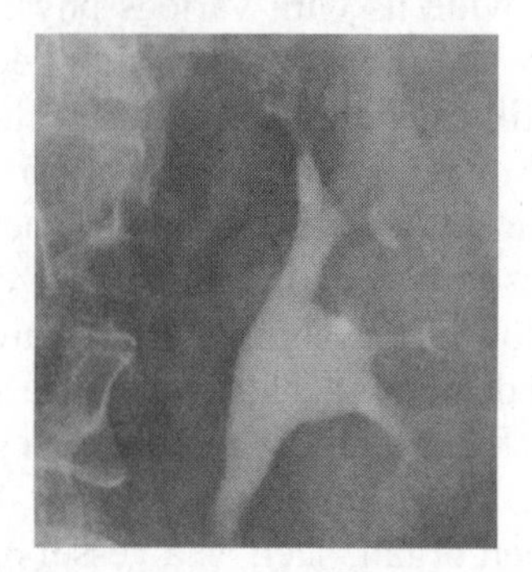

Fig. 1.5. Urography image

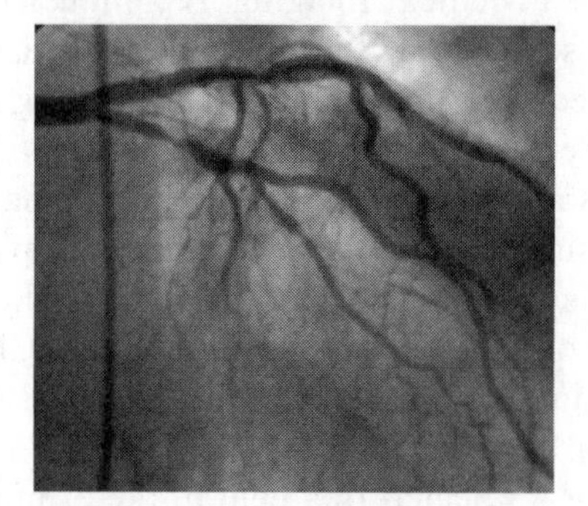

Fig. 1.6. Coronarography image

When necessary, an image of the large portion of the human body can be obtained (X-ray of the chest – Fig. 1.7). Making use of the fact that different tissues will absorb different amounts of X ray energy, the images are obtained which are not generated in simple physical processes but reconstructed by way of computations.

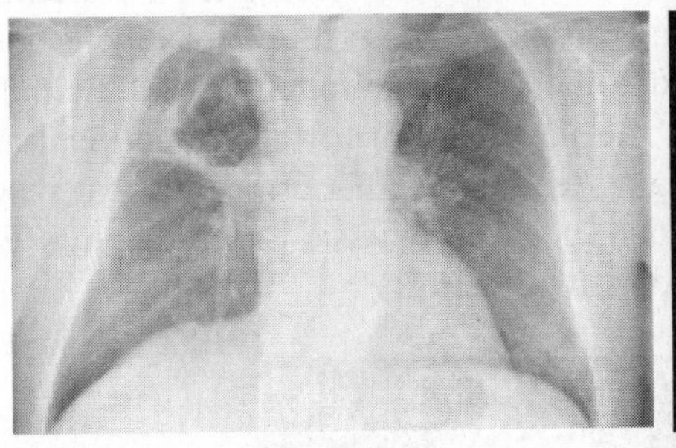

Fig. 1.7. X ray image of the chest

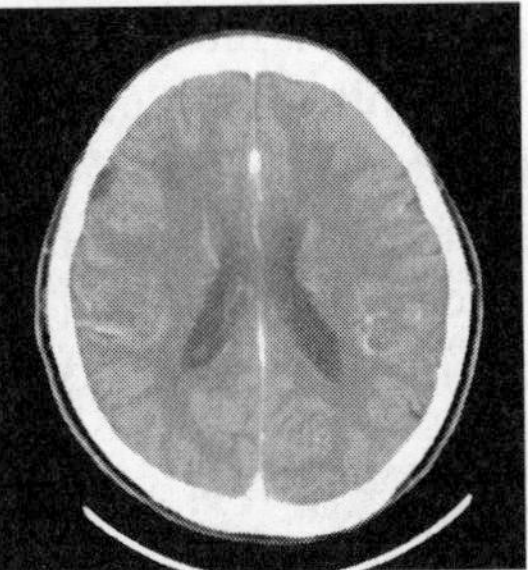

Fig. 1.8. CT image of the brain

The technique of computer tomography CT (Fig. 1.8) is often used here and it involves precise measurements of the total amount of X-radiation absorbed along several lines passing through the patient's body at various points and at various inclinations, yielding the matrix of quantities that, after visualisation, provide the cross-sectional images of the patient's body also in those parts where classical X-ray images are mostly useless since the vital biological structures, where the differences in X-ray absorption capacity are very subtle, are nearly wholly obscured by a structure being a strong absorbent of X-radiation (as in the example of very delicate brain structures hidden by massive skull bones – Fig. 1.9).

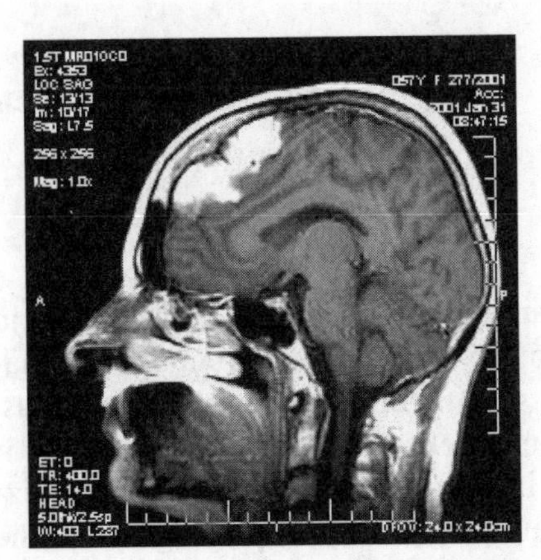

Fig. 1.9. Brain structures hidden by massive skull bones

The method of image reconstruction on the basis of collected and duly processed physical signals was first applied in X-ray tomography. Now medical imaging uses various physical processes involving the differentiation between body tissues depending on their density as well as their other properties, and this allows us to combine the image mapping and the morphology of the body organs with the information on their functional aspects. These methods include imaging techniques that utilise nuclear magnetic resonance NMR (Fig. 1.10) and, positron emission tomography PET (Fig. 1.11), SPECT (Fig. 1.12) and many others.

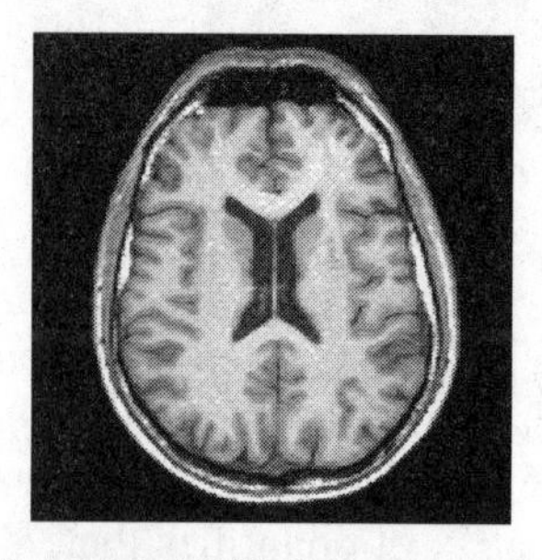

Fig. 1.10. NMR image

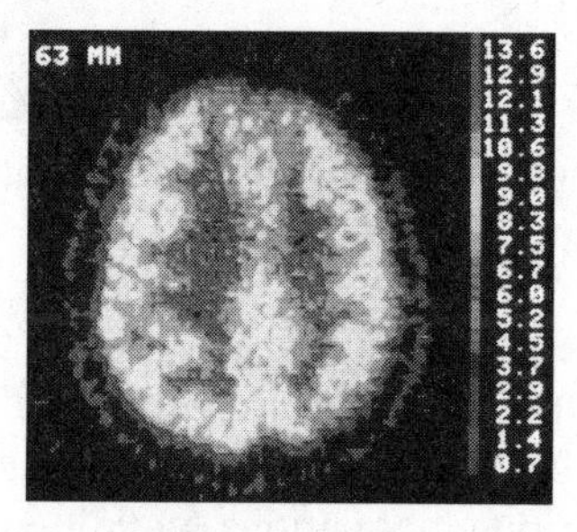

Fig. 1.11. PET image

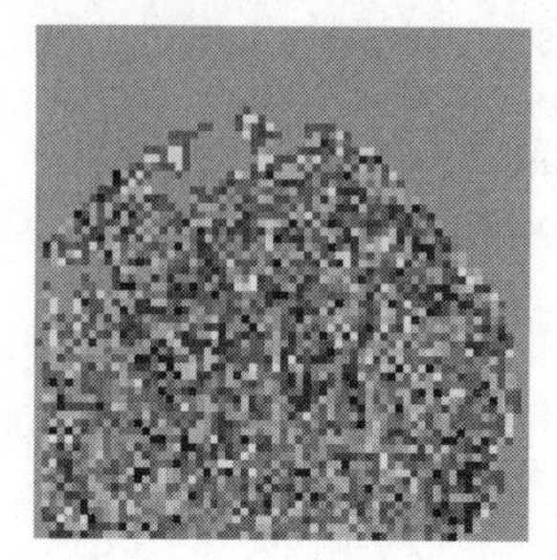

Fig. 1.12. SPECT image of the heart

The physical agent used to penetrate the insides of the human body in order to obtain the required medical image may have different physical nature, and hence can be adapted to the specific applications and conditions. Well-known imaging techniques, not mentioned previously, include: ultrasonography USG (Fig. 1.13) yielding images organs and tissues and utilizing the absorption and reflection of ultrasound waves passing inside the body and received by a special receptor head.

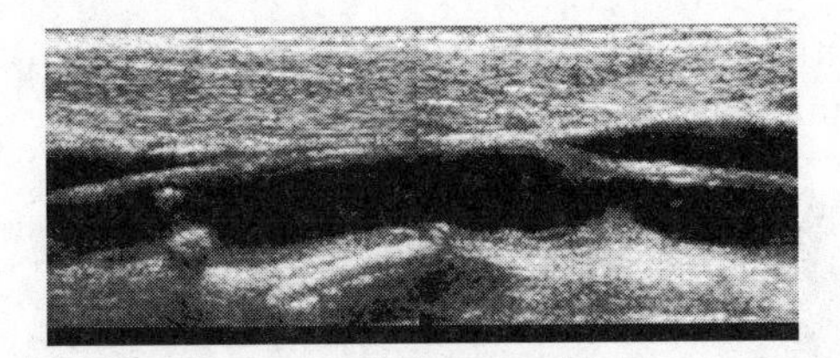

Fig. 1.13. USG image of the left common carotid artery

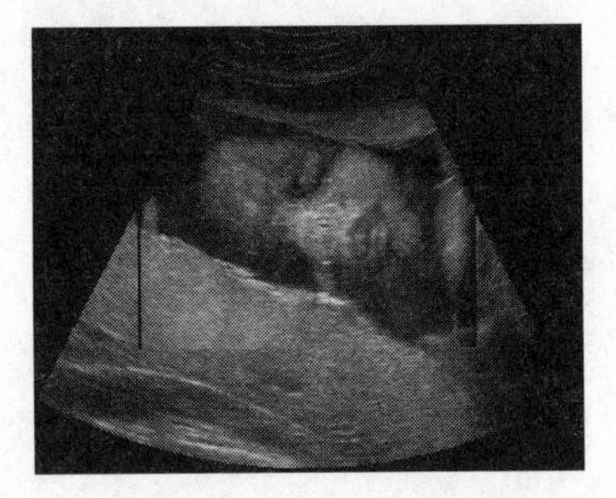

Fig. 1.14. USG image of foetus inside the uterus

The way in which these waves are represented is such that even the most delicate structures can be imaged (such as a foetus inside the uterus Fig. 1.14 or removable artificial heart valves). One of the major advantages of USG is that it allows for the detection of structures which could not be otherwise imaged (for example textural changes visible in USG images, revealing different mechanical properties of tissues having the same chemical composition, allowing for the detection of cancerous lesions in the liver - not seen in X-ray images – Fig. 1.15). Another advantage of this method is that it is nearly non-intrusive; hence the examined structures (even the most delicate and vulnerable ones such as unborn babies) can be subjected to uninterrupted and long-term observations while the patient does not suffer any ill effects.

The agent penetrating the interior of the human body in USG imaging is a multidirectional beam of emitted ultrasounds and the method makes use of the mechanical properties of the body tissues (as they affect the speed of ultrasound wave propagation within the patient's body and are responsible for wave reflection, refraction, dispersion and attenuation). Other physical agents can also be used to penetrate the human body, such as weak electric currents, yielding images portraying the distribution of impedance of body tissues – which may also prove valuable. New advancements in bio-impedance techniques seem more promising and might become a mine of valuable information supplementing the data obtained now with the use of currently available imaging techniques.

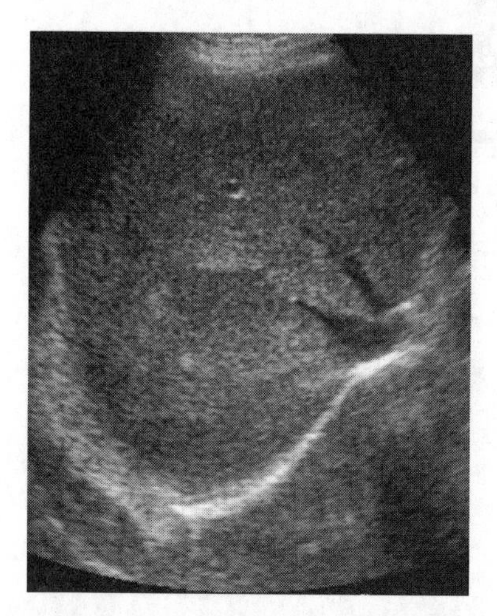

Fig. 1.15. USG image showing cancerous lesions in the liver (Image courtesy of MedPix, Uniformed Service University)

Autoradiography techniques offer different possibilities than the methods mentioned above. These methods consist of the visualisation of ionising radiation (usually gamma radiation) emitted by radioactive organs. Undoubtedly these methods are intrusive as a precisely measured amount of a selected radioactive isotope (for instance iodine in thyroid gland examination) has to be introduced into the patient's body, preferably in the form a chemical compound which easily enters the metabolism processes and which are actively absorbed or removed from the organs that need to be examined. Through the analysis of the topographic distribution of the internal sources of radiation: i.e. the atoms of radioactive isotopes contained in the chemical compound temporarily integrated in the structure of the examined organ, we obtain a 'map' of the metabolically active areas (hot and cold spots/tumours) – Fig. 1.16, which is an excellent basis for a precise and reliable diagnosis. Because the process of metabolic reaction of isotope-marked compounds is dynamic (i.e. time-variant) and observations of changes in radioactivity with the use of imaging devices (gamma cameras) do not enhance the level of invasiveness of examinations (even those lasting for a long time). Therefore, one can not only trace the actual shapes of examined organs, but can also follow their time-variant functioning, which is the most valuable source of information.

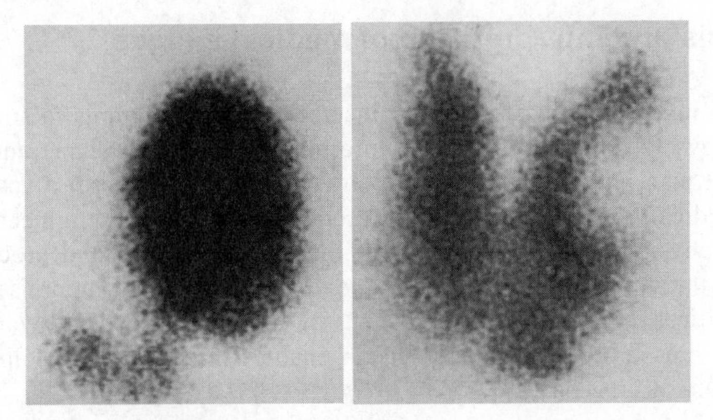

Fig. 1.16.a–b. Autoradiography images of hot and cold tumours

A specific type of radiation associated with the functioning of living organs is infrared emission due to the fact that metabolic processes usually lead to the production and dispersion of heat. It has been a well-established fact for over 20 years that thermo-vision images are a mine of valuable information on the structure and functioning of some parts of human body, for example in enabling us to observe the blood flow in tiny blood vessels on the body surface, invisible with an unaided eye, and to diagnose certain illnesses (such as breast cancer). Hence methods using thermo-vision should be added to the long list of the most useful medical imaging techniques.

All these images provide physicians with vast and valuable information and often serve as one of the major premises in the process of formulating diagnosis, prospects and current therapy or rehabilitation control, since the human being – a visualiser, tends to refer to the analysis of images when faced with a **difficult** problem-solving task. Undoubtedly, medical problems belong to the group of difficult decision-making processes; hence it is not surprising that the whole system of medical education, as well as the generally adopted methods of medical diagnosis will refer directly or indirectly to images. Physicians tend to support their decisions on a visualised morphology of organs or the use of various forms of artificial imaging (i.e. PET or spectroscopy in NMR) to present functional aspects of the examined organs or their parts.

1.2. Analysis and interpretation of medical images

Thanks to the inventiveness of many engineers' and their attempts to still find better ways to collect and present information about the shape and functioning of man's internal organs, we now have at our disposal a vast number of medical imaging techniques. Present-day bio-medical engineering provides physicians with all images of the internal organs and processes; and furthermore it gives them the tool for improvement, appraisal and the classification of images: computer vision- an advanced IT technique. At the present stage computer vision enables three types of computer processing of images:

- *image processing* – aimed **to improve the quality** of the image (enhancement, sharping and contrasting) and to separate and highlight only those **objects** which are vital from the medical point of view (segmentation)
- *image analysis* – aimed to determine the features of the whole image or specified objects, to count the objects and compute the value of quantitative parameters **or names of categories** assigned to quality features
- *pattern recognition (or pattern recognition*) – aimed to identify and classify the highlighted elements or areas through indexing them as objects belonging to certain categories determined a priori- mainly on the basis of their shape, dimensions and texture.

The relationships between the considered techniques of medical image processing are shown schematically in Fig. 1.17. The classical computer vision techniques will be described very briefly as there are numerous books and other publications on the subject. Besides, selected issues will be also addressed in Chapter 2 of this book. One has to bear in mind that all of these three steps of classical computer processing of medical images are becoming more widespread, which clearly shows their major role in biomedical engineering. These techniques prove to be particularly useful tools for medical physicians as thanks to image processing and enhancement the details of the examined organs and processes are brought to light, which helps them to provide a reliable diagnosis. Having at their disposal computer results of analyses of image features and objects, physicians may support their reasoning on more tangible and reliable premises than just visual image evaluation, which improves their efficiency and gives them the feeling of confidence and security. Finally, more and more widespread techniques of automatic recognition and classification of highlighted biological structures may help the physicians to provide the right diagnosis though they sometimes require a critical approach to automatically suggested categorization as each pattern recognition technique admits a certain level of error. Physicians, on the other hand, are never free from personal responsibility for their decisions.

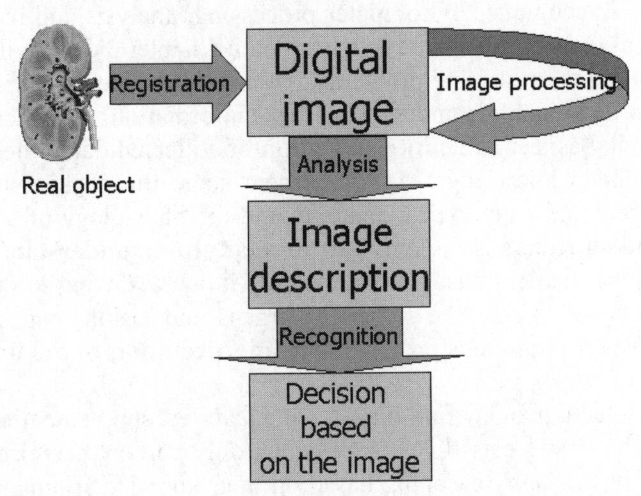

Fig. 1.17. Interrelations between the classical components of image processing

But there are some problems in this model of co-operation between 'computer vision engineers and the physician because of the still insufficient development of proper methods for automatic interpretation of medical images. This task is very difficult because of two types of troubles:

- First, the morphology of the health organ is different for every human being, so we do not have any kind of template (or pattern) of the 'proper view' of the analysed object.
- Second, deformations of the organ shape and size can be very different in form, number and also in localization if the diseases are in fact identical!

This problem will be discussed more detail in the later chapters of this book, but at this moment we can point out the proposed solution of the problem under consideration: We need a new mechanism for the application of contemporary computers for medical image utilization for physicians' purposes. This mechanism needs to be connected with the merit content of medical images instead of its form. We have proposed and developed such a mechanism and have called it the 'automatic understanding' of medical images. We have dedicated this entire book to the description of this concept and its application.

1.3. What new values can add to this scheme 'automatic understanding'?

All afore mentioned techniques of computer processing, analysis and recognition of medical images (discussed in more detail Chapter 3) prove insufficient to tackle all the tasks and problems that arise in connection with the use of images as valuable sources of medical information. The most fundamental and vital aspect is the **interpretation** of collected data, referring to the physician's knowledge. At the present stage the physicians' knowledge of correct and pathological anatomy and the physiology of examined organs and structures is the only key to their proper **understanding,** and this why the medical image looks the way it does. Owing to the computer processing of images the shapes of organs and lesions can be better visible; however physicians provide their **interpretation** of the image.

The process of selection and definition of image features, supplementing the automatic analysis and classification provides only certain **premises** for the process of physicians' reasoning based on their knowledge, imagination and sometimes also intuition. Without a meritorious interpretation of the results of all analyses and elements of automatic classification, they become useless for the purpose of diagnosis and therapy; the actual values of specified image parameters or the categorization of imaged objects are of minor importance. One thing that is important for the physician (and the patient of course): what does this all imply in terms of patient's condition, the suggested diagnosis of an illness, the optimal therapy or rehabilitation and the chances for success? Contemporary techniques providing various types of medical images (briefly summarized in section 1.1) as well as IT technologies including computer vision depend on one major factor: the **interpretation** of medical images by humans (i.e. well-qualified physicians).

The process, however, is becoming increasingly difficult for humans (i.e. physicians) as the numerous and complex images made available to us by technological advancements require that physicians acquire new skills and qualifications to correctly interpret them and it usually takes longer than the development of new technologies. Furthermore, new imaging techniques provide the physician giving the diagnosis not only with one image as before, but with many (sometimes more then ten) images taken for one patient that have to be analysed. These numerous images portray, for example, subsequent cross-sections of the brain tissue obtained with the use of tomography or present the organ at various stages of the process of absorption or removal of the chemical agent. Sometimes the same organ can be observed with the use of several imaging techniques. Thus the diagnostic procedure becomes more detailed and reliable though, at the same time, however, it requires extra effort on the part of physicians.

As the analysis of such a number of different images is becoming increasingly difficult and time-consuming, a physician may overlook a lesion visible in one of the images only, which in consequence may lead to an error in the diagnosis. Besides, we can hardly expect that a physician will be able to analyse and evaluate all available medical images as there are so many of them and the visual forms of the presented organs may differ too, depending on the applied imaging technique. Further complications result from the fact that a physician has in fact no time to become accustomed with all forms and shapes of images since new-generation medical apparatuses are entering the market at a fast pace. In the past physicians found routine a great help: at a first glance an experienced radiologist would pinpoint the part of the image which required his particular attention and then ignore other morphological details, visible but not important. Nowadays physicians are not able to acquire such a routine as medical apparatuses are now always being replaced with newer, improved versions and physicians are not given an opportunity to become accustomed with them. Renowned (and rather rich) hospitals which try to catch up with the technological advancements and attempt to acquire the newest diagnostic apparatus are now faced with a major problem. The apparatus are better, there is more information available and yet the physicians feel somewhat lost: before an image provided by one of the diagnostic systems becomes as familiar to them as a dial-plate of the clock, new –generation equipment will appear and well-known images will be replaced with new ones: maybe better and more refined but unfamiliar.

When we consider in this short summary of problems associated with the interpretation of presently available medical images, how many organs can be examined and how many types of deformations and lesions are possible, we should not be surprised by the statement that this branch urgently needs the strong support of advanced IT technologies. Actually as new techniques of medical imaging are developed, there is a growing demand for better techniques of computer-assisted analysis, interpretation, classification and recognition of available medical images. People tend to expect that modern equipment will not only portray the interiors of the human body and give it a maximally clear representation, but will also perform the preliminary analysis of the thus obtained image directing the physicians' attention to those elements which may carry the most vital information for the diagnosis. This means that the computer has to make a (sometimes complex) computation of the value of each of several million pixels making up the image. Furthermore, it is expected to perform an intelligent analysis and pass on suggestions to physicians – this is a major challenge for IT engineers who must not only develop but also constantly improve imaging techniques. This book is the result of several years' of work of the Authors, who developed and tested several methods for assisting the **meritorious interpretation** of medical images, which involved going 'deep inside' the image contents. In light of the main concept presented in this book, two basic assumptions have to be made. The first assumption is that a semantically-oriented (linguistic) description of the medical image contents can be created automatically, which is exclusively on the basis of duly performed analysis of graphic structures detected in the image and their interrelations. As a rule, such analysis ought to be preceded by preliminary image processing, involving the carefully chosen sequences of routine procedures of image filtering, segmentation and transformations so that the components vital for image interpretation are brought to light while technical distortions and factors responsible for biological variety are eliminated as they may hinder the semantically-oriented analysis. The other assumption is that a semantically-oriented description of the medical image contents, vital for diagnostic purposes, ought to be confronted with the appropriately expressed **semantic expectations** and predictions (in our case those included in the graph grammar). These semantic expectations are derived from our knowledge a priori about the diagnostic and prognostic meaning of certain structures contained in the considered class of medical images; hence they are specific for the given field. This means that a proper representation of knowledge, which is the key to an automatic understanding of medical images, **is not** universal and has to be generated separately for each category of medical problems. In other words, a proper representation of medical knowledge (for instance in the form of graph grammar) is required for each type of medical imaging, for each organ and disease. Undoubtedly, this is long and hard work, but when completed, **automatic understanding** of a wider range of medical images can be made possible. This should prove to be a strong incentive for the further development of medical imaging techniques, particularly in the field of medical image **interpretation** which so far has received little attention, thus the classical triad: processing, analysis and recognition of medical images can be extended and/or strengthened.

The dependences and relationships between the 'traditional triad' of computer vision techniques and the new approach given by means of the automatic understanding of images can summarized as in Table 1.1.

Table 1.1 Relationships between the computer vision techniques

Stage of image utilization	Question answered in the traditional approach	Question answered in the new (proposed) approach
Image processing	How to increase the quality and visibility of the image?	What follows the visualised details?
Image analysis	What are the exact values of selected features of the image?	What is the meaning of the features extracted from the image?
Image recognition	To which classes (patterns) do the selected objects on the image belong?	What are the results of the fact that some objects belong to particular classes?

Technically speaking, the difference between pattern recognition and image understanding includes the following assumptions:

- in the case of recognition we always have a fixed number of a priori known classes and the task only demands the extraction of all these image features, which are necessary and sufficient for the differentiation between classes under consideration. After processing we obtain the number (or name) of the proper class;
- in the case of understanding we do not have any a priori known classes or templates, because in fact the potential number of possible classes goes to infinity. So after processing we obtain a description of the image content without using any a priori known classification, because even the criteria of classification are constructed and developed during the automatic reasoning process.

Now we try to explain, who and when can use such an approach in the wide field of medical images.

1.4. Areas of applications for the automatic understanding of images

1.4.1. T-formed area of applications for the automatic understanding of medical images

The technique of image understanding described in later chapters has only just come into being and will be developing for some time in all areas and zones of application, as new manners of use, which we do not know and cannot expect, will be discovered. However, it may be stated that this technique will have several very interesting applications which are worthy of the efforts put into its development. Now, we will show and analyse three types of **T**-formed areas of the application (Fig. 1.18).

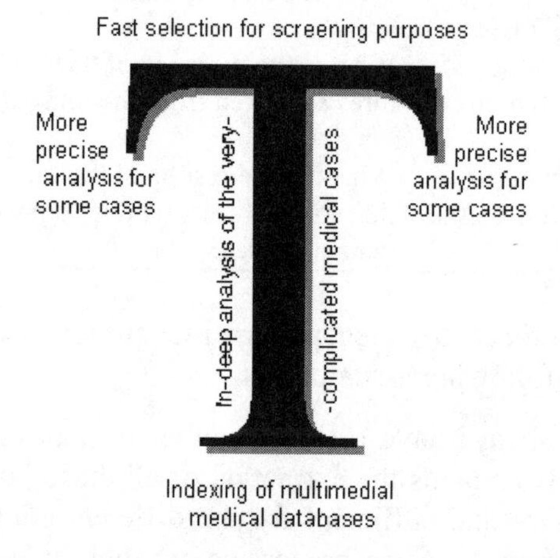

Fig. 1.18. Symbolic structure and abbreviated characteristics of areas of application for the automatic understanding of medical images

The upper part of the considered diagram consists of the area of population investigation. With the type of application characterised in subsection 1.4.2., the tasks of a computer capable of **image understanding** require the analysis of a large number of graphical data – this area of applications is symbolised by the top dash of the letter T, because the range of analysis is **wide**, and the **depth** of analysis is rather small. In certain cases we may perform a deeper analysis, as shown in the drawing and discussed in subsection 1.4.2.

The other area of application of the automatic image understanding technique is deep and requires a detailed analysis of particularly difficult images, especially in case of doubts and difficulties in deciding on final diagnosis. In such cases, a computer well equipped with automatic image understanding programs as described in this book may support a diagnostician analysing subtle and hardly visible features to improve the conformity of the diagnosis (calculated as the average of many examined cases). Certainly, such an ambitious target may only be reached in relation to a narrow area of the problems, hence the symbolic structure of application of automatic image understanding methods illustrated in Fig. 1.18 reflects the discussed problems with a part of the letter T characterised by a very small width and at the same time going deep into the problems under consideration. The more detailed characteristics of this task are described in subsection 1.4.3.

Furthermore, a more detailed area of the problems connected with a part of the T letter, usually called a 'sheriff' located at the base of the letter symbolises the opportunities connected with the application of automatic image understanding to semantic indexation (oriented to the meaning not to the form!) of multimedia, medical data bases. This problem requires a more extensive introduction for improved understanding and will be discussed further in subsection 1.4.4. Here, we only note that one of the far-reaching advantages of automatic image understanding is the possibility of overcoming the problem of finding meritoriously (and not only formally) adequate records in multimedia, medical data bases. The automatic image understanding technique will allow users to search for records on the Internet (and also in other image and multimedia resources) based on meritorious criteria (i.e. related to similar types of pathology) and not on superficial similarity of medical images. In subsection 1.4.4 we will show that automatic image understanding will allow the automatic indexation of numerous medical data bases which are extremely difficult to search (because they are so numerous!) and that the same technique may significantly facilitate the automatic questioning of information systems and to obtain the required information with a very narrow margin of wrong or inadequate answers.

Having described above the general application of the automatic image understanding technique we will now try to characterize it in the following subsections. We will concentrate mainly on what we need, not what we may reach, because this part of the book is devoted to asking questions, and only subsequent chapters of the book are devoted to the solving of problems.

1.4.2. The Automatic understanding of medical images as a tool for the preliminary classification of imaging screening data

The first area of application for automatic image understanding is through the use of a computer as a tool for the preliminary analysis and selection of a large number of diagnostic images obtained during population investigations. This refers to the upper part of the already mentioned 'T' letter. The role of automatic image understanding in the cases considered in this book is concentrated on the sensible detection and indication of all images containing disturbing symptoms in patients whose cases require thorough analysis. The role of an intelligent or well-designed computer program is that of the 'preliminary filter' in extracting a small number of interesting cases which are hidden in the ocean of trivial cases, and may be extremely useful in the screening of large populations (Fig. 1.19).

Population screening is very expensive, as it requires thousands of images for the targeted population (i.e. school children, all workers of a given organization, all people living in a given region, etc.). However, screening is worth it and is advisable. It is also interesting from an economic point of view, as such screening is much cheaper than the treatment of patients with advanced diseases, even if we do not take into account the individual and social suffering connected with the late detection of diseases, long time treatment, and the numerous failures that often end in the death of a patient. Furthermore, population screening is now practically feasible, because modern diagnostic systems are more easily accessible and more effective. For instance, and as we already know, 1st generation scanners needed between 5 and 10 minutes for one CT result, but modern 5th generation scanners require milliseconds. Therefore it is technically feasible and more viable economically to obtain a larger volume of data in a very short time, including good quality medical imaging for hundreds of thousands of people.

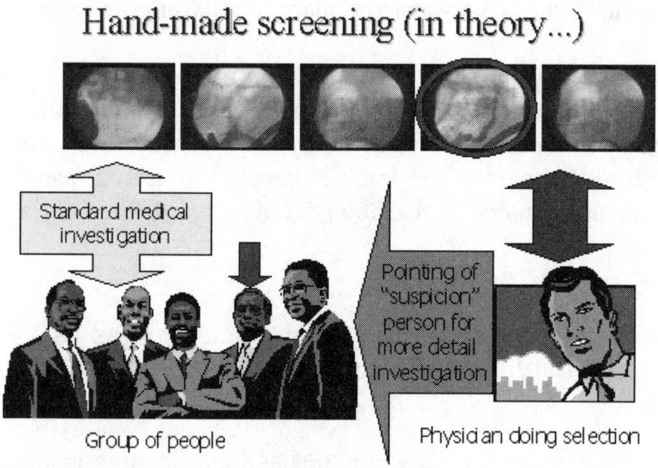

Fig. 1.19. Theoretical model of 'hand made' screening

An example of a very well-known type of medical image screening is given in Fig.1.20.

It should be underlined that present-day screening is related to the prophylaxis and the early detection of cancer and other dangerous diseases, since early detection (at the stage when symptoms are imperceptible for a patient) is the key for successful treatment.

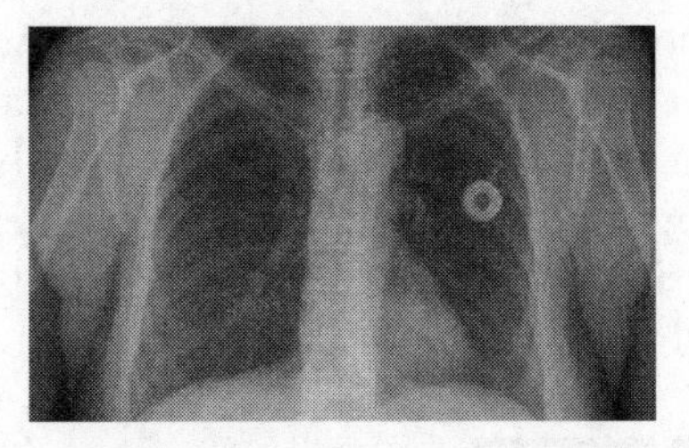

Fig. 1.20. RTG image of the chest as a much known example of medical imaging for screening purposes

However, analysing such a large collection of diagnostic materials is a real bottleneck. It should be added, that in focusing purely on medical images, we may argue that even the best qualified and most industrious practitioner is able to analyse less than a hundred images per hour. What is more, the majority of such images would illustrate cases with no pathological features, and a doctor may become bored and could lose concentration due to specifically understood mental, though not sensory, deprivation. Consequently, when an image containing early, not visible at first sight, but noticeable symptoms of a disease, it is possible that a doctor will treat them as images of a healthy person – usually it will end with fatal consequences for the patient whose disease has not been spotted (Fig. 1.21.). Such incidents may bring the whole idea of screening into question.

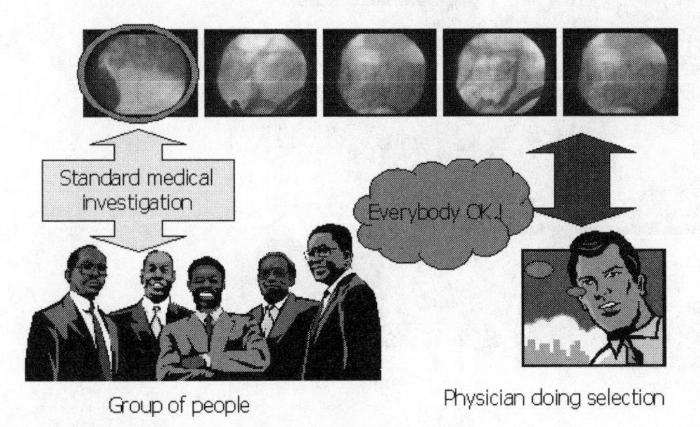

Fig. 1.21. Mistakes in 'hand made' screening

In this situation one should really consider employing a more modern computer technique, such as the automatic image understanding technique described in this book (Fig. 1.22). Although it is already well known we would like to emphasize once again that automatic imaging analysis is always carried out with the same precision and that a well constructed analysis program will always detect pathological symptoms, even the frailest ones, regardless of how many boring, trivial images it has had to analyse before. This feature is worth striving for!

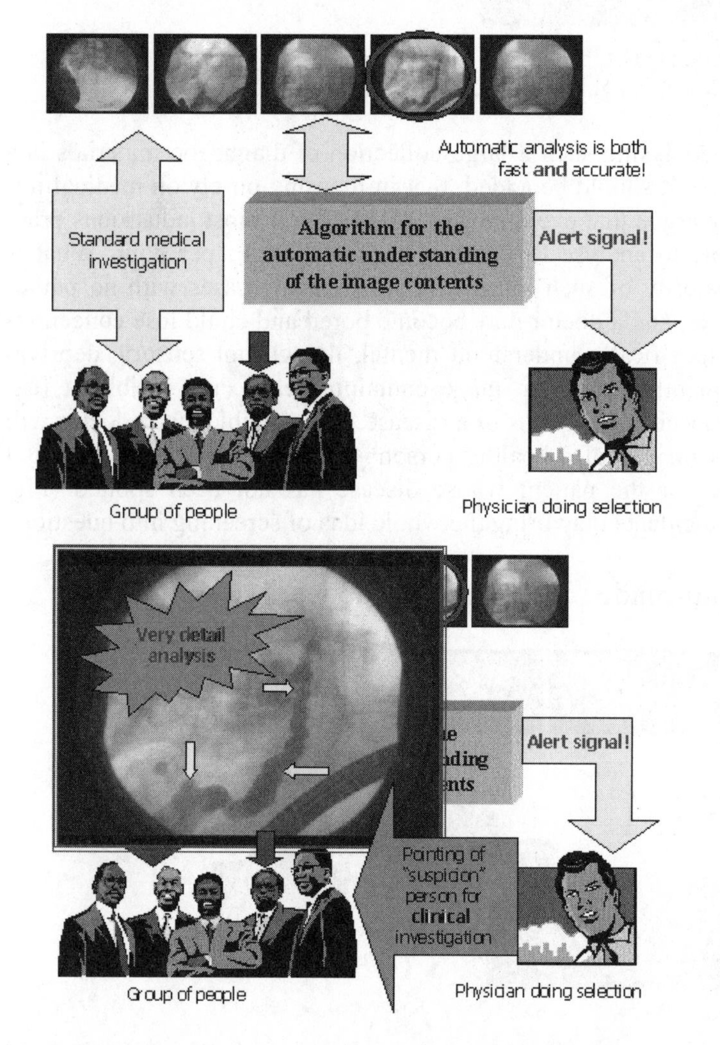

Fig. 1.22. Automatic system, which helps the physician in screening (selection of the 'suspicion' data and aided by computer analysis)

The most important task for the computer visual system is the **pre-selection** of registered images (Fig. 1.22 upper part) because it is extremely difficult for human beings to extract important diagnostic information from numerous and diversified images, even when we do not take into consideration the large number of images showing tissues and structures **free** from any pathological symptoms. After selecting the 'suspicion' data, the automatic system can also help the physician in the deep analysis of image details under consideration (Fig. 1.22 bottom part) – but this is in fact a not so important part of the job. The most important goal for the automatic understanding system is connected with the generation of 'alert signals' in the area of application.

The above described selective tasks seem easy, just a simple dychotomic classification – whether images are normal or whether they reveal a kind of pathology. In fact, this task is very difficult and sophisticated, and the source of difficulty is in the expression 'a kind of'. The automation of a very sophisticated diagnostic task is easier when we know what we are looking for. And in the case of screening images are selected without knowing what we are looking for within them – and that is the source of problems (Fig. 1.23).

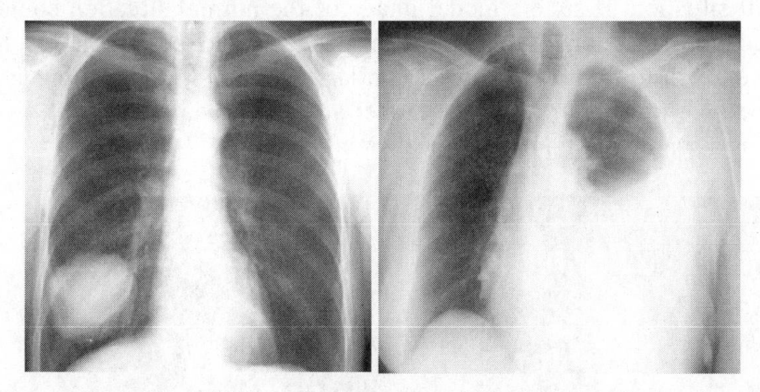

Fig. 1.23.a–b. Two different RTG images of the chest showing various forms of the same pathology (tumours) (Image courtesy of MedPix, Uniformed Service University)

We will now consider these details for a moment because this is characteristic for the whole field of automatic medical image understanding, and it is worth discussing this in the context of selected, screened population images. In this case, a computer has to draw the attention of the doctor to an image that reveals that something is 'wrong'. It is, of course, impossible to predict what should be searched for, as pathological symptoms may appear in various organs visualised at the same time (screening usually employs medical images showing vast fragments of the body, for example, the chest, the abdomen, etc.). What is more, pathological changes may appear in various parts of the organs, they may have different shapes, sizes and properties – in a word, and although absolutely unpredictable they should be detectable.

We can also imagine a different situation in tasks connected with computerized early hazard detection systems (i.e. for technical diagnostic, military, property protection purposes, etc.). In such cases we do not know the form of hazard to be detected, but we are able to describe the **lack** of one (for example, rhythmic operation of a jet engine, no visible intruders at the attended area, etc.), so instead of detecting hazards we are able to recognise the safe state and detect a situation when the state of safety is no longer recognizable.

Medical problems are more complicated, as a **normal** image of the examined organs and other elements of the human body are almost as unpredictable as an image of the searched pathology. The essence of the problem is that each human being is different and, in a sense, unique, so it is practically impossible to define something that may be called a model of the normal situation. If such a model image of the normal situation could be defined, the selection of screening images would be simple, as it would be enough to find a measure of similarity for each analysed image, so as to be able to compare it to the model and treat each significant discrepancy as a synonym of a pathological situation (Fig. 1.24).

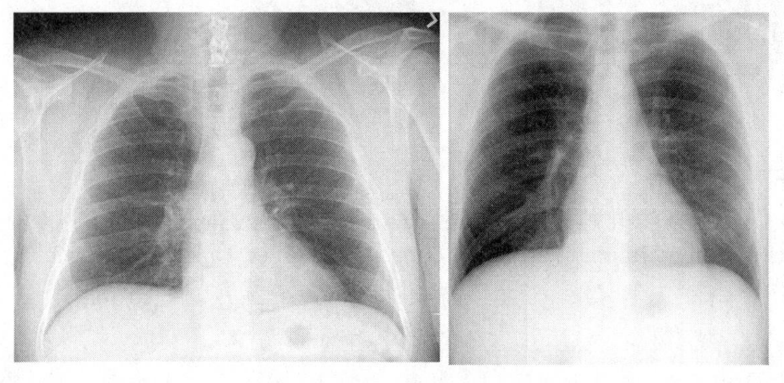

Fig. 1.24.a–b. Two different RTG images of the chest showing various forms of normal cases (Image courtesy of MedPix, Uniformed Service University)

As indicated above, a simple classification pattern for screening images based on the 'health model' recognition cannot be applied the same as it is impossible to define a universal pattern of pathology. It is therefore not possible to have such images automatically allocated to certain, relevant categories (normal image or pathology suspected) on the basis of a conventional *computer vision* technique. In such circumstances it is advisable to look for a different method, and this should begin with the question: How does a practitioner cope with a given classification and a computer not? The answer is obvious. A practitioner looking at the image, visualizing human organs tries to understand why they appear as they do, and which biological reasons cause a given shape, shadow, brightening, or other details – hence, doctors not only see the image but they also see what starts a complicated and very often unrealisable, mental process which originated in their skills and experience. If a computer has to perform something similar, then we would want it to perform a reasonable classification of the images and this may be achieved on the basis of automatic **understanding** of what is visible in the image. If we could only design the computer to neglect a form of the image and bring out the content (employing the methods described in this book), we would achieve the required effect.

Consequently, it is necessary to create the basics of the automatic, medical, image understanding technique in the context of all tasks connected with the automatic analysis of population screening images, as it is the only way to arrive at the conclusion of what is normal and what is dubious. If a computer could give (with below described methods) meritorious evaluation of the considered image confirming that its content does not show any pathological features, then such image may be archived without further inspection by a doctor. Thanks to such mechanism (if invented and implemented), outstanding medical specialists, experts in evaluation of medical images will save a lot of time as they will not have to view and analyse trivial cases. However, if automatic interpretation of the meritorious sense of the image indicates any features of pathology, a doctor must evaluate such image. Of course, sometimes 'suspicions' formulated by the computer program understanding the sense of the investigated image will not be confirmed by a doctor, but despite such errors application of such program will be positive. First, as it has been mentioned above, this program will significantly reduce the number of images, doctors have to deal with, and second, the doctor's attention will be mobilized and directed to the image of any pathology signalled by the computer (with clear indication of location and character of the pathology).

Two risks are connected with the application of medical image automatic understanding programs as a tool for the selection of screening results. First, the program may have parameters set in such a way, that it becomes 'over-suspicious'. If this is the case, the program will not be very useful as it will send a lot of unwanted images to the doctor for consultation. On the other hand, however, even a single case of automatic elimination of an ill person's image, thereby avoiding consultation, creates an unnecessary and dramatic situation which should not be allowed. Therefore it is necessary to reach compromise solutions, though it is not easy in the case of automatic image understanding, because ROCs may be very difficult to construct for the purposes of the discussed methods.

It is widely known however, that each classification method may separately estimate the sensibility and specificity of methods, and these parameters are interrelated, so an increase in one parameter causes a worsening of the other. Therefore, it is necessary to find a criterion, for instance, as given:

Assuming that the real percentage of incidents of a given disease in the whole screened population is 2%, we may say that the operation of a selected program is reasonable providing that it identifies and sends the doctor 20% of the total number of viewed images including **all** incidents of real pathology. If the program enables the doctor to verify 80% of the images, or by mistake, the program eliminates even 0.01% images of persons who are really ill, then such a program is practically useless.

The introduction of **three** (not two) categories which constitute the answer obtained from the image understanding system may help to overcome problems of seeking a compromise between sensitivity and specificity. The first category consists of images with no traces of pathology; such images should be archived as they may be useful for tracing back in case the same patient is examined again. The second category consists of images directed to a doctor because the program has found certain symptoms classified as pathological ones.

The third category consists of images which have neither a positive nor negative 'opinion expressed by the program'. A doctor must obtain such images for review, as an expert opinion is always decisive, specifically when the automatic recognition of the image ends in failure. However, the third category requires the marking of images in such a way that a doctor is not alarmed by tricky suspicion, but he knows that there is a problem, and a patient should be re-examined. Such problems may appear in case the imaging is incorrectly performed and contains artefacts that make interpretation difficult.

1.4.3. Automatic understanding in difficult medical problems

The above described task of employing a computer system equipped with automatic medical image understanding only for the pre-selection of 'suspicious' images in screening results from practical reasons. Disease prevention and preventive medicine becomes a very important medical field in all advanced societies. This gives rise to some specific requirements and expectations connected also with equipping medical sciences with technical means and, in particular, it leads to a formulation of new scientific tasks whose objective is to create new information systems supporting physicians involved in preventive treatment and preventive medicine. These tasks can be considered priority ones, especially in view of the currently on-going demographic processes, in which we are dealing with the ageing of whole societies, especially in developed countries. A growing number of elderly people result in that increasingly large parts of population **require** screening medical examinations. This is due to the fact that elderly people become increasingly more prone to various diseases; among these diseases are also such diseases which can and should be detected early in population screening (this is true particularly for neoplasm, cardiac and cardiovascular system diseases). There are no doubts that a computer can be used as a tool enhancing significantly the efficiency of relevant preventive examinations. This is especially important in this field, in which these examinations face serious obstacles, i.e. in the field of interpretation of collected data, and in particular in semantic analysis of recorded images.

However, if we take into consideration that for this task we want to employ the most sophisticated technique of artificial intelligence, which in this book we dare to call automatic image understanding, we could express our doubts whether the task of automatic scanning the screening images is sufficiently ambitious if we compare it to the complexity level of the tool designed for the task. Although in the previous chapter it was proven that supporting the work of a medical doctor performing a preliminary analysis of the collected screening data requires the use of this new technique (that is understanding and not only recognition of images), otherwise no reasonable selection could be performed. Still, this task had a frustrating element to it resulting, for example, in a very arduous penetration of the semantic content of an image, and after overcoming many difficulties and obstacles, the computer was able only to classify an image as correct or **possibly** as a pathological one (this was the only thing required from it). Certainly, in some selected cases the suggestion given to a physician by a computer **could** include additional information (as indicated at the ends of the T-letter bar in Fig. 1.18), which conveyed what the software detected in the examined image owing to that it was adapted to automatic image understanding. This, however, was rather a side effect.

We cannot expect more from this task, at least not at the present stage of information technology development. In the situation of massive work resulting from screening examinations, the variety of possible pathologies is so huge that leaving the final decision to the computer would be too risky. This is why in this task the entire advanced decision-taking process connected with image assessment and with diagnosing a patient must stay in the hands of a medical doctor and there is nothing to change it.

A different and scientifically more interesting situation arises when from the start we narrow down the application field of the developed automatic image understanding algorithm to selected specialist problems (even very difficult ones). If we locate the considered computer system in a clinical hospital of a given specialisation (i.e. cardiology or gastroenterology clinic), we **know** its field of operation because patients admitted to the clinic have been already diagnosed and are seriously ill. While building a computer system designed for an intelligent image analysis for the needs of a defined clinic, we may take two assumptions that will significantly narrow down the task but it is precisely this that allows us to apply a deeper analysis process.

First, we may be sure that the image to be analysed certainly **contains a form of pathology**. A healthy person, for instance, pretending to be ill or a hypochondriac would not be admitted to the clinic at all because the fictional character of his/her illness would be properly detected and interpreted by a practitioner without whose recommendation the patient could not be admitted to the hospital. Exceptions to this rule should be picked out by the medical staff of the clinic (among others based on their long years of experience gained due to extremely frequent contacts with patients suffering from some defined types of diseases). This is why a person mistakenly referred to a clinic should be discharged from it before complicated and expensive diagnostic procedures, whose element is also the automatic image understanding considered here, have been started.

Secondly, a disease that we are trying to recognise automatically (using automatic understanding of medical images of various types) indisputably concerns a defined organ of a patient and no other part of his/her body. This assumption is based on the generally accepted hospitalisation system, which places patients with cardiological diseases separately from those suffering from neurological or urological problems, etc. That is why when analysing medical images in a given clinic we can assume *a priori* with high a high degree of probability that they will show cases of patients whose problems are connected closely with one type of disease of a strictly defined organ, which simplifies the analysis significantly.

As results from the above, a computer system used to medical image analysis in a clinic has a more narrow field of operation in comparison to the system discussed in the previous subsection in the context of screening data selection. Hence, the 'leg' of the T-letter is so narrow. On the other hand, however, usually these are extremely difficult cases (also in the diagnostic sense) because simple and easy cases are treated in ordinary hospitals rather than in clinics. Therefore in order to diagnose it is necessary to perform a thorough and careful analysis of all data concerning the diagnosed patient, including all obtained medical images. Usually diagnoses must be performed in atypical situations or a very subtle differentiation between numbers of *a priori* equally probable diagnostic hypotheses must be made. It is precisely due to this fact that clinical problems require a thorough analysis. They are symbolised by a part of the T, which reaches deep down and reaches fundamental decisions and assessments based on an in-depth analysis of very small, hidden or hardly detectable image features (Fig. 1.25).

Here we arrive at the fundamental question of whether any computer software will ever able to penetrate the semantic content of an analysed medical image **better** than the eye and mind of an experienced specialist.

Please note that the task to which computer scientists assigned themselves is very ambitious and at the same time difficult; it is much more difficult than the task described in the previous subsection. In the task analysed earlier it was enough for the software to manage images **not worse** than any medical doctor would have to contend with. It did not have to be better (we even assumed that it stood no chances of being better) but the software had the strength to analyse all images with equal attentiveness. These features of automatic image understanding demonstrate its purpose, ability and usefulness in screening examinations: as a tool for the initial sorting of many images from numerous patients, without the need to expose humans (a medical doctor) to a boring and frustrating analysis of such a 'mass' of images. A task defined in this way, as we said in the previous chapter, could be solved with the use of the computer image understanding technique.

Can the same be said about the advanced analysis of highly specialised images, with which we are dealing in advanced clinical examinations?

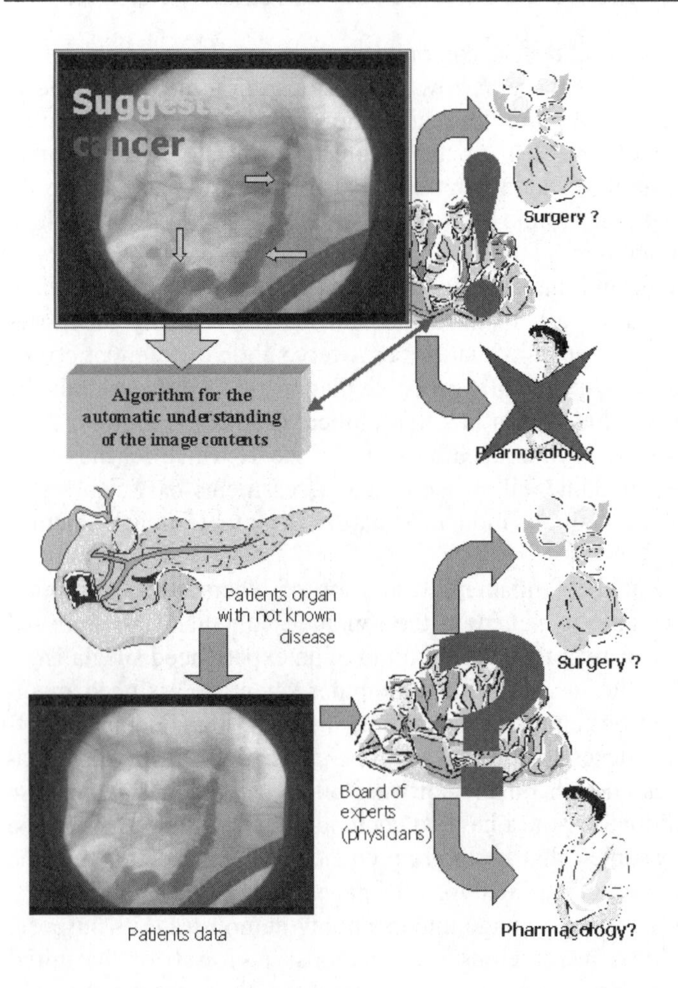

Fig. 1.25. Assistance from the 'automatic image understanding system' in difficult diagnostic problems

The problem is indisputably more difficult, because in this case we cannot take full advantage of a computer's speed and at the same time expect it to perform all analyses with the same (maximal for its capacity) care and attention. Clinical doctors, as opposed to physicians reviewing population-screening images usually do not have to hurry because they usually deal with a small number of patients. These doctors know that only the most difficult cases were addressed by the clinic and that their treatment is an especially responsible task; this is why they try to devote their best will and knowledge to all of their patients. If computers are to prove their usefulness in this case, it is necessary to put a lot more effort into the construction of a system that can understand the contents of recognised images when there is a need to 'compete' against the human skills in a situation, in which the technique has no advantage resulting from a simple comparison of the operational speed of a computer and of the human being.

However, one **can** undertake the above characterised task and it is worthwhile to strive for the possible success, although it is unquestionably more difficult. Let us indicate these features of automatic image understanding that may constitute strong points in direct competition against medical doctors in the tasks of such difficult specialist diagnostics at the level of advanced clinical examinations.

Computer technology can determine some subtle object features with greater precision and thus supply the options necessary to differentiate more finely difficult and complex cases than would be assessed by physicians 'at sight'. Automatic image understanding allows reference to numerous quantitative features determinable in images, such as sizes and the spacing of various elements, integrated or averaging optical density of various fields, values of their area surface, the length of the edge line etc. The doctor's eye when analysing an X-ray image (or any other medical image) looks consciously or unconsciously for these parameters and bases his/her reasoning process on them. Here the computer has the upper hand since it can detect deviations from the correct parameters much faster and more precisely than it is possible to achieve by visual inspection. What is more, computer image analysis enables reference to such object features which are practically impossible to detect by means of visual image inspection, as for example, the degree of irregularity or curvature of particular contours, angles between lines determined in various ways (for instance the symmetry axis) on the image. These also include the enormous number of more advanced graphic features such as various proportions, geometrical moments, shape invariants, etc. These features carry sometimes considerable significance.

Let us consider an actual example originating from examinations with the use of the computer tomography method (CT). As it is well known, the symmetry of both presented parts of the brain (i.e. both brain cerebral hemispheres) is very important for the evaluation of CT and MR images. A doctor is as good as the computer in noticing and evaluating large asymmetries of analysed biological structures (Fig. 1.26) but in case of small asymmetries, human eye finds it difficult to detect that one side of the image prevails over the other (in a way, of course!). On the other hand, a computer can do it very precisely, locating the pathology that has more seriously disturbed the symmetry of the image (Fig. 1.27).

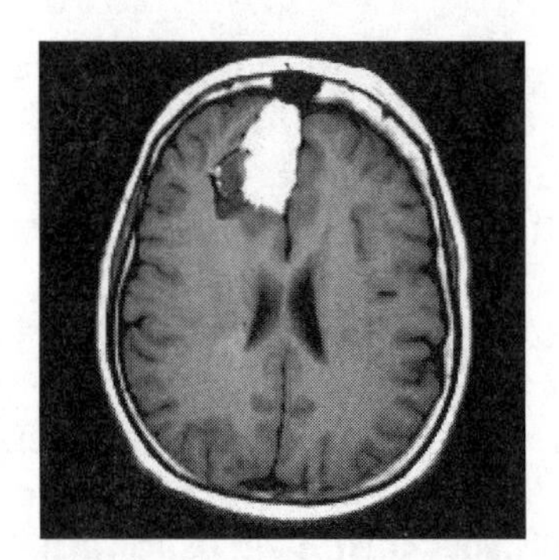

Fig. 1.26. CT image with a well visible asymmetry in brain structures

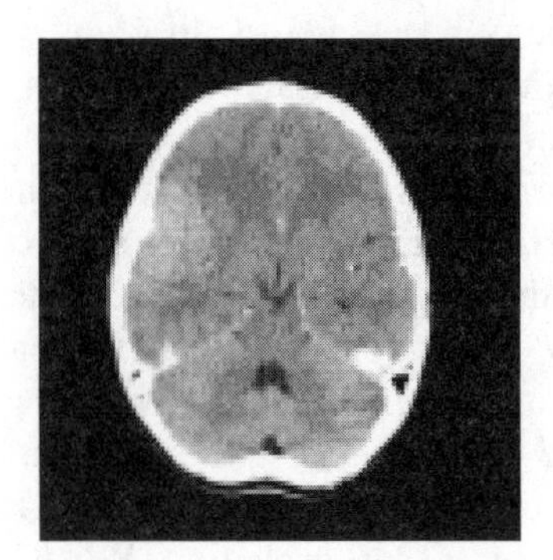

Fig. 1.27. CT image with small asymmetry (lesions) in brain structures

As a result a computer is also more precise (and beyond comparison more repetitive) than a human being in classifying image elements to relevant categories. This results in a significant improvement of the **stability** of computer-constructed diagnostic procedures, compared to those that a medical doctor could propose. Let us use another example from the research performed by the authors. Investigating the methods of computer processing of ERCP images (*Endoscopic Retrograde Cholangio-Pancreatography*) we have found out that the presence (or absence) of lateral ramifications of the visualised pancreatic duct is a very significant element of the diagnostic procedure. In the case of a healthy pancreas such ramifications do not exist; in the case of an advanced pathology the edge line of the visualised duct is often very irregular. It is important, however, whether the discovered disturbance of the duct's regular contour can be classified into the lateral ramifications category (which could be considered to be a symptom of chronic pancreatitis, Fig. 1.28) or whether it is a cyst, which is a neoplasm symptom (Fig. 1.29). Classification is not difficult when we consider obvious cases, such as those shown in the figures, but when pathological forms with ambiguous shapes occur, pathologies are difficult to classify (see Fig. 1.30).

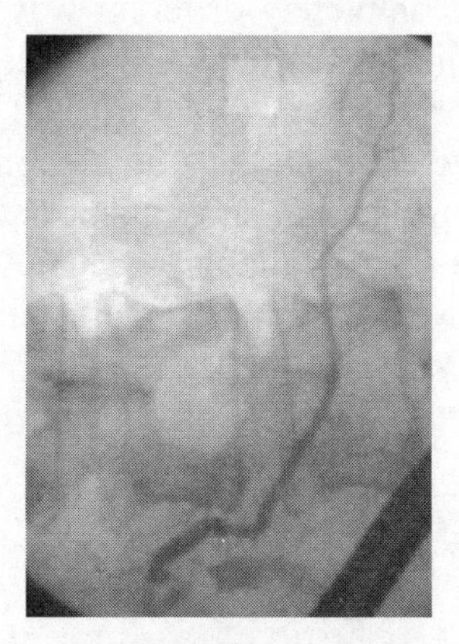

Fig. 1.28. ERCP image with symptoms of chronic pancreatitis

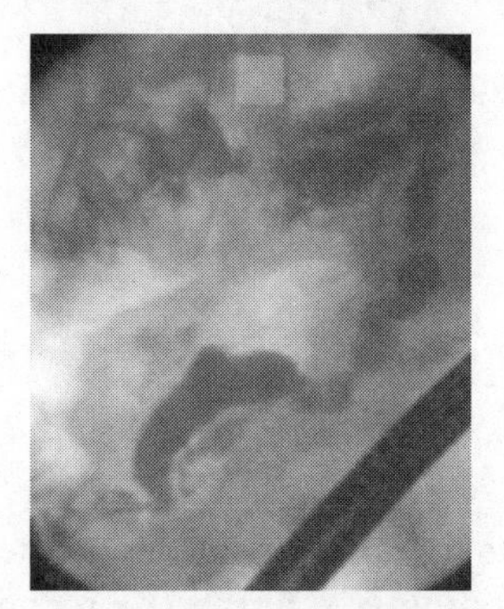

Fig. 1.29. ERCP image with symptoms of cancer of the pancreas

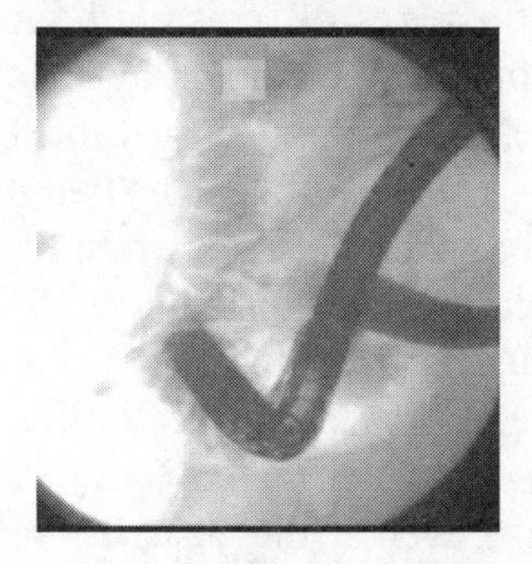

Fig. 1.30. ERCP image with symptoms difficult and ambiguous to diagnose

In such cases a physician has to make an arbitrary decision on his/her own. This can result in, that in various circumstances the same (or very similar) geometrical form will be classified in completely different ways. Owing to the technique developed by the authors for the objective resolution of doubts whether ramifications are real or apparent (see Fig. 1.31), the decision is taken on the basis of an objective criterion that can be continuously optimised (on the grounds of comparisons with subsequent data coming from next patients whose ERCP images are available and whose diagnosis has been verified by a performed surgery). What is more, this criterion is certainly repeatable and unambiguous.

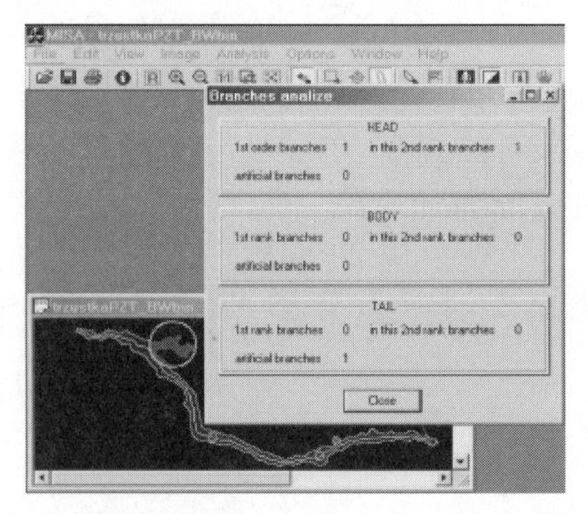

Fig. 1.31. Verification methods for real ramifications in pancreatic ducts

There are big opportunities to gain an advantage in the field of computer medical image understanding owing to the computer's ability to reconstruct, by means of computation, a collective three-dimensional model of the examined organ (or its part) on the basis of a series of registered two-dimensional images. In this way we can reconstruct spatial images for practically any organ (Fig. 1.32) but in this case, the computer's advantage in **interpretation** of these images becomes even more noticeable. People enjoy looking at three-dimensional reconstructions like those shown in Fig. 1.32 but they find it difficult to assess the similarities and differences. We need not look very far for examples: it is enough to mention that we are able to see quite precisely (if we have been adequately trained) the differences in the proportions of surfaces of plane figures. Yet recognising proportions of solid figures is much more difficult, even if the visualisation system allows the virtual 'inspection' of a digitally reconstructed object in different (simulated) illumination and to see the figure from various sides.

A computer is able to calculate just as easily and use the parameters of a three-dimensional structure of on object, as those that it determined on plane images; thus gaining the upper hand.

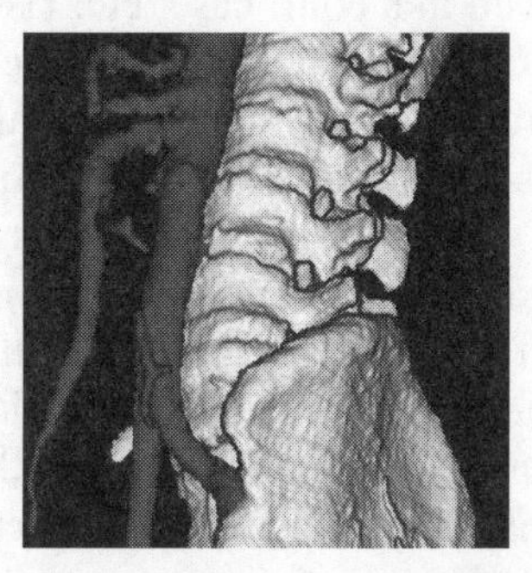

Fig. 1.32. 3D reconstruction of the abdomen aorta
(Image courtesy of MedPix, Uniformed Service University)

Obviously, the problem could be understood like this: different methods of digital image analysis provide various parameters characterising the image to be used by a computer equipped with software for automatic interpretation of these data. Such software, having access to a great number of data necessary to take the decision can 'beat' a physician. But this does not authorise us, regardless of its advancement, to call it an automatic image understanding system. All these parameters calculated by the machine during the analysis of an image could be also used by a medical doctor and then we would see who is better at diagnosing!

The above reasoning is wrong because it does not consider an additional issue concerning the psychological nature, which reduces the intellectual advantage (indisputable and never questioned) of a physician over a computer. The discussed issue is a problem with taking a decision when there are numerous features supporting differing arguments and, as a result, decisions. A computer applying relevant methods (described in further sections of this book) can take a diagnostic decision considering, in an equal and balanced manner, so many data that we are not able to collect. In fact, the more data the better because the decision will be better justified. On the other hand, humans facing the need to take a decision in the presence of very numerous data, each of which influences the decision somehow, feel uneasy and in extreme cases, they are lost to such an extent that become unable to do anything at all. This is true not only about a physician confronted with dozens of results of various analyses and examinations of one patient. A director of a bank choosing a business strategy on the basis of hundreds macro- and microeconomic factors is in a similar psychological trap, and so is a politician stormed with arguments of proponents and opponents of a given solution. No different is the situation of a judge considering contradictory arguments of parties involved in a court case, etc. Usually, people forced to take decisions in such cases select just a few arguments (practically, no more than seven) from a large number of available data. These few arguments form the basis for further reasoning while others are in fact not taken into consideration. If the choice of the basis is correct, the decision taken can be very good indeed. After all we are all familiar with examples of wise decisions taken by people in difficult situations. However, this is not always the case when among the data on which the decision is based there no some clearly dominating ones, and when the correct action should be a combination of many small factors considered simultaneously, the result of the decision taken may be far from optimal. Businessmen and military men have known about it for a long time and they use advisory computer systems willingly.

All the above arguments are aimed at showing that complex and difficult diagnostic problems arise. Therefore if a lot of symptoms can influence the decision (which can be found by a computer images analysis) it would be advisable to take the next step and associate the advanced computer image technique with relevant AI methods. This would be done so in order to automate the remaining process to the same extent as the data collection process has been automated. This postulate is best implemented by the technique of automatic image understanding described in this book.

To close this chapter let us say why, in the described diagnosing tasks of complex and difficult medical problems based on some specified medical images, we believe it to be necessary to relate to the above-mentioned new term **'image understanding'**, rather than sticking to the well known and successful term of **image recognition**.

Fascinated by the facility with which IT systems operate on digital images (which owing to specialist medical devices or digitalised cameras can be easily transferred to the computer and subsequently, using simple software, stored, transmitted, processed, printed, etc.) we often believe too quickly that we can make use of image information as easily as we can of figures and text. But we are wrong. IT at its current stage of development can easily master the **form** of an image but the **content** remains completely inaccessible for the field of automation. All the processes concerning the practical application of visual information – among others, in medical systems – and seemingly simpler search processes for image information on a given topic in large multimedia data bases, highlight drastically the fact that in the case of an image (contrary to figures or text), the **form** of information can be in fact only loosely connected with its **content**.

In particular it often happens that images **different in their graphic form** carry **the same content**. This is illustrated in Fig. 1.33 showing the same medical problem in the form of two completely dissimilar images registered in two different patients but leading to the same diagnosis.

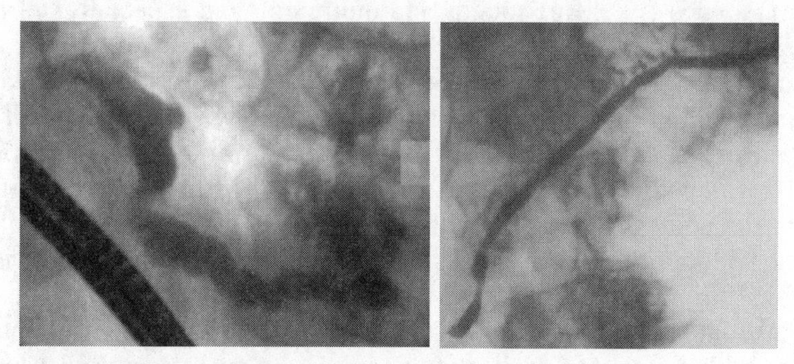

Fig. 1.33.a–b. Both ERCPs show pancreatic cancer but the images are not that similar to each other

Since the form of an image is not identical to its content, we need tools which will allow us to 'extract' the content (semantic sense) of the image trapped in its more complicated form. **Automatic image understanding** postulated by the authors both in this book and in other publications consist of automatic extraction of some significant sense, which **is** contained in the image but trapped in its form. The fact that the content is trapped in a complicated form of the image means that the content is not easily visible on the image but that it requires special mental effort to bring the sense out and to **understand** it correctly.

1.4.4. Automatic understanding of images as a tool for semantic searching in data bases and successful web crawling

The tool described in this book, i.e. a set of automatic medical image understanding methods, can be applied in one more way, symbolically connected with the lower bar of the T letter (see Fig. 1.18). A need for this application results from the fact that IT resources stored and processed in IT medical systems become, to a growing degree, multimedia resources. They consist not only of text information, which are normally collected and looked up in all data bases (in the case of medical data bases such typical data are: patient's particulars, epicrisis, description of diagnostic and therapeutic procedures, case record, etc.) and, apart from easily computer-processed numerical data (i.e. results of physical measurements and biochemical analyses) also various signals. To be more exact we could indicate that the above-mentioned non-alphanumeric medical data stored and analysed during medical examinations as well as during on-going treatment of patients, are various bioelectric signals (ECG, EEG, EMG, ERG, ENG, etc.), sounds (i.e. heart sounds and murmurs), and especially, various images.

A characteristic feature of these signals (registration of various information is semantically not reducible to a text or a set of digits, especially medical images) is, among others, that in general their **ontologies** have not been well developed yet; therefore in semantic networks they are very difficult from the point of view of intelligent **servicing.** However, as has already been said, multimedia resources of medical information collected in the numerical form keep growing and this growth will continue to accelerate if we take into consideration the planned development of telemedicine. Difficulties with the use of such multimedia data may be analysed from various points of view but we shall focus on the problem of search techniques, in particular on **semantic** search important for medical sciences, i.e. one concentrated on its meaning content. This can be very troublesome because if there is no exact (and competently prepared) verbal description accompanying it, it can be difficult to find multimedia information meeting some defined criteria, if based only on the form of the registered signal (for example, based uniquely on the image bitmap). This is the very place where we could inform about another application of the automatic image understanding technique described in this book and treat it as a tool for intelligent indexation.

Let us imagine that we have resources of medical images collected on digital carriers but deprived of detailed semantic description. This assumption is fully justified in reference to most hospital data bases known to the authors, as well as enormous and still growing resources of medical images collected and made available in the Internet. In such a case finding an image illustrating a chosen, pre-defined problem (e.g. in order to illustrate a lecture) can turn out to be extremely difficult, and in extreme cases it can mean that we have to search once again through a large number of images (after their time-consuming, therefore expensive, downloading from the web) until we find the right one. The situation is even more difficult when we want to see **all** available images with **the same content meaning** (e.g. the data of all patients with identically located and similarly advanced neoplasm as is the case of a patient currently treated). Such needs are quite frequent, since the method of checking the type of therapy applied to other patients (and its consequences) is one of the most popular paradigms used for therapy selection. Yet searching multimedia data bases to find the meaningful content of images remains a task practically unsolved.

In the above-described situation the concept of automatic image understanding discussed in this book creates very interesting possibilities. If we had an effective tool, which by analysing just the medical image, could assign automatically to this image its semantic description, we could use the following procedure. A computer equipped with an automatic image understanding software views systematically the available medical multimedia data bases and tries 'to understand' the content of each image. Of course, this task should be a background task and performed only when there are no new commands from the user. Upon this review, for some images located in data bases, it will be possible to create their semantic descriptions automatically (their content will be understandable for a computer as a result of automatic analysis). If the semantic meaning of an automatically analysed image, together with its record ID containing such a 'decoded' image is found out, the image is linked to the record containing the whole 'deducted' semantic description of the image (Fig. 1.34).

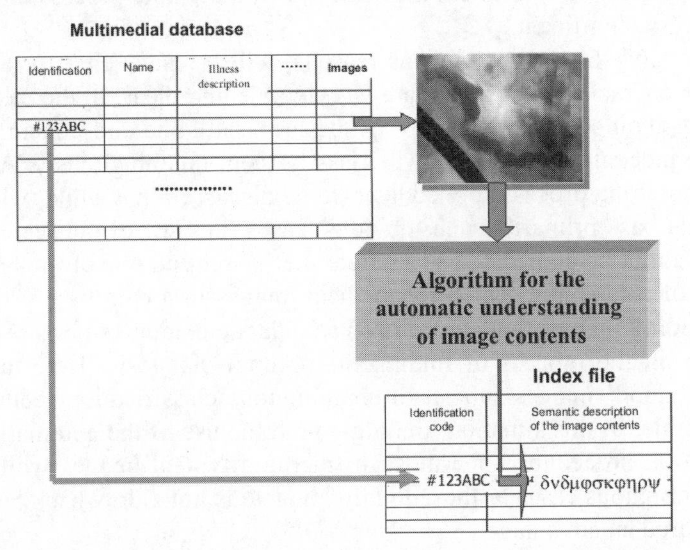

Fig. 1.34. Automatic image understanding for the indexation of the multimedia data base

This description usually consists of a series of symbols denoting the semantic content of the image in an unambiguous way, even though usually illegible and incomprehensible for a human (hence to mark them on images we use Greek letters). Principles governing the creation of such descriptions and their methods of operation will be described later in this book. For the time being we shall only mention that the technique that will be used for this purpose will be based on methods of mathematical linguistics using specially constructed graph grammars.

An automatically generated semantic description should be located in a special index file of the computer, which scans the base. The description itself should always be located outside the data base due to the fact that in no situation should the original data base be 'littered' (automatically generated semantic descriptions of an image can contain errors!). Moreover, searching through separate index files is much faster than searching through the whole base 'pumped' with large volume digital image records. A relevant record should appear in the index file for each image for which (as a result of automatic semantic analysis) the code representing its meaning is discovered. The share of images understandable for the computer can vary; probably it will take a very long time before it is be possible to build such an efficient semantic indexation mechanism, which would be able to find an adequate description to each medical image from any data base. However, taking into account the objective of the whole process, this defect is not very significant.

An effective indexation, for obvious reasons, will be made first for all images whose characteristic features are very legible and clear. In the case of such images their semantic analysis will be successful and consequently the automatic indexation procedure will classify them unambiguously. As a result, the searching process applied later (to be discussed in a while) will find in the data base primarily such 'obvious' cases; in view of the search purpose this cannot be considered as a defect. Let us remind ourselves that the objective of a semantic search for medical images in a data base usually means finding images that can be used as didactic examples or as reference objects in the process of finding the optimal diagnosis. Here the usefulness of 'good' images subject to unambiguous classification seems to be indisputable. In this situation, finding – with the use of the automatic image indexation procedure – the most distinct and typical images while leaving out ambiguous cases or those highly atypical is not a drawback but can be considered an advantage.

The only problem (if any) can be that as a result of such indexation not all objects from the data base will be indexed. For some of them, that is for those that turn out to be too difficult for the automatic understanding procedure, there will be no automatically assigned semantic description of their content. Of course, it will not be possible as a result to use them in the automatic reasoning process. However, if the data base is rich enough (and the analysed technique is introduced precisely because data bases have recently grown to very significant sizes), then after the process of automatic indexation there will be so many identified (that is available for use) records that in applications requiring calling them, we shall not face the problem of deficit.

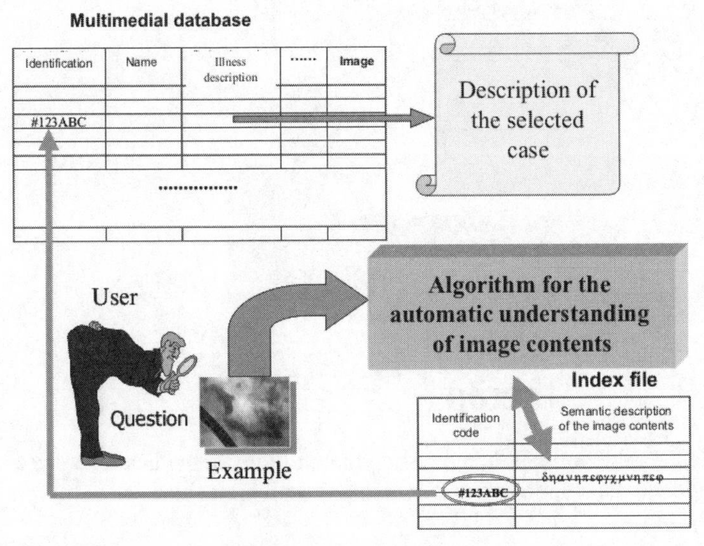

Fig. 1.35. Context-related search for the required information in a semantically indexed multimedia data base.

Let us show now how to make use of a semantically indexed multimedia data base when we need information on a given subject. Let us assume that a query submitted to the considered data base has also the form of an image *('show me something similar to..... ')*.The sequence of actions taken is presented in Fig. 1.35. First, an image exemplifying the object of interest (constituting the basic part of the query to the data base) is subjected to the same procedure determining its meaningful content, as the procedure used for the data base indexation. A code (analogical to the code used for the base indexation) developed as a result of the attempted **automatic understanding** of the image meaning content allows one to find in the index file all these items whose automatically generated description shows a defined degree of similarity to the code of the image given in the search query. Based on the knowledge of identifiers of medical records corresponding to these items of the index file in indexed data bases, it is possible to extract the required information and to use it in accordance with plans

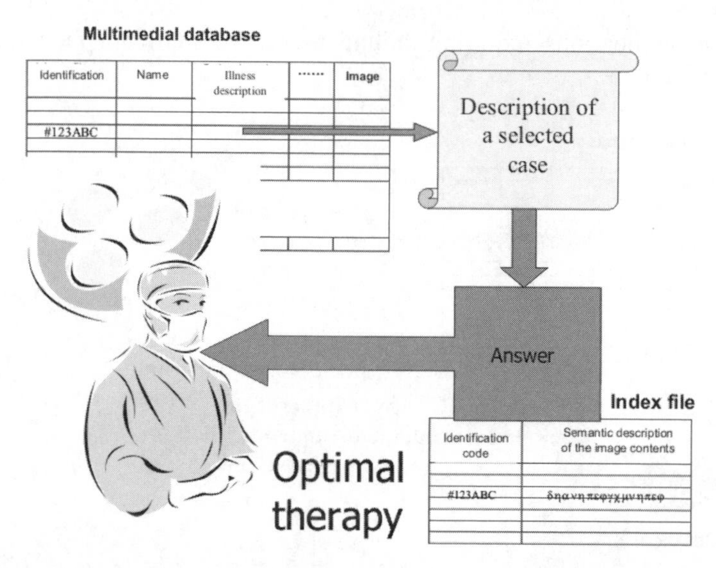

Fig. 1.36. Selecting the optimal therapy using the multimedia medical data base and the intelligent (based on image understanding) search machine

The above-described mechanism of indexation and the semantic search for the needed medical images can be organised pursuant to two schemes. The first one is designed for the data base client. In this pattern, the above-described indexation of objects in data bases and conversions of queries submitted to data bases, as described in this book in the semantic form, take place in the client's computer. In other words a user who foresees that he/she will want to access in a semantically oriented way any information resources, recommends to his/her computer to carry out an indexation of relevant data bases. The indexation is run according to the pattern shown in Fig. 1.34. However, it must be taken into consideration that the data base is located on a server (sometimes very distant one) and the tool for image intelligent understanding and the index file created by this tool are on the client's computer. The strength of this approach is that it can be implemented at any time by any user who has access to the scanned data base and who has a tool for automatic understanding of the image content. Its disadvantage is the high indexation cost resulting from the fact that in this solution practically every image contained in data base must be transmitted via the web to the client's computer; there an attempt at its content understanding is made. In a situation in which a number of clients of the same server want to use the same system to enhance their work, the very same work (very time-consuming!) will be repeated unnecessarily many times.

Indexation performed by the owner of the data base is a complementary solution. In this case the automatic image understanding software must be located both on the server (for continuous indexation of the data base, which, of course, keeps changing its content all the time) and in the client's computer (to convert images displayed during queries).

2. A General Description of the Fundamental Ideas Behind Automatic Image Understanding

2.1. Fundamental assumptions

In this chapter we shall try to explain what automatic image understanding is and how we can force the computer to understand the image content. Before we get down to details we must demonstrate that there is in fact a fundamental difference between a formal description of an image (typically obtained by means of a variety of computer viewing methods) and the content meaning of the image, which can be discovered by an intelligent entity, capable of understanding the profound sense of the image in question. Although the problem under consideration is rather serious, we shall now use a joke to show how weak traditional computer vision technology can be in applications in which image understanding is the bottleneck of the proper solution.

The joke goes as follows: Imagine, that we have a big multimedia data base and that we are trying to find a picture 'telling the same story', as pictures serving us as our specimens. Examples of such images are presented on Fig. 2.1.

Let us combine our thoughts as to how we can describe the criteria for an intelligent selection of other pictures from a multimedia data base, similar (with regards to their semantic content) to the ones shown on Fig. 2.1.?

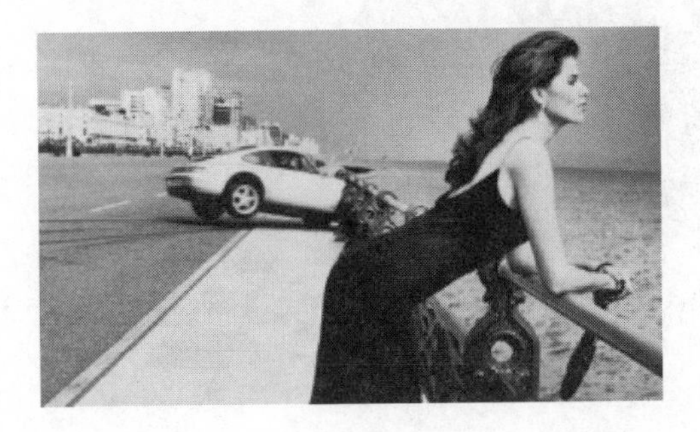

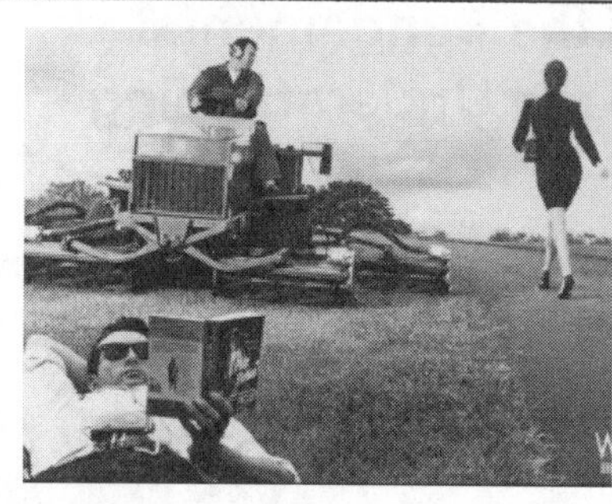
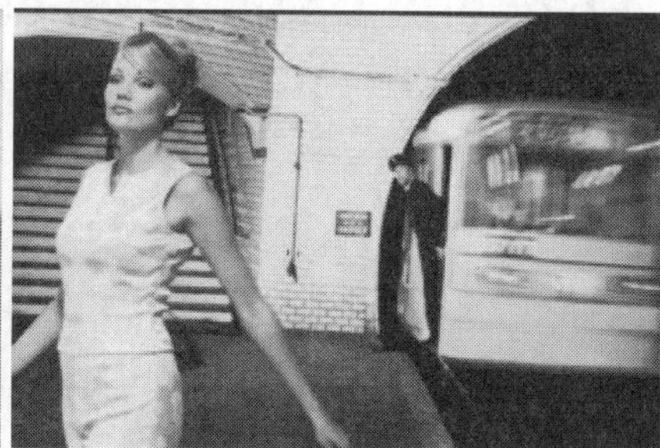

Fig. 2.1.a–c. Examples of images

To solve this problem using a classical image analysis one needs the following operations:

- Segmentation of all pictures and a selection of important objects in all images
- Extraction and calculation of the main features of the selected objects
- Object classification and recognition
- Selection of features and classes of the recognised objects which are the same on all images under consideration
- Searching in a data base for images depicting the same objects, with the same features

Executing the steps specified above on the first image under consideration, we find elements highlighted on Fig. 2.2.

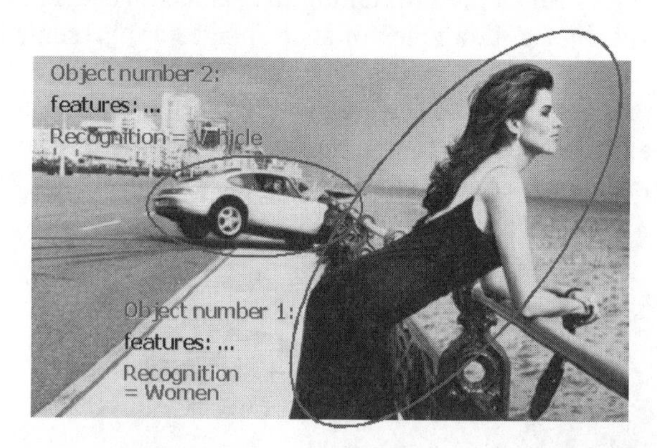

Fig. 2.2. Results of a formal analysis and classification applied to the first image under consideration

A similar analysis can be performed for other examples of images (we shall skip the figures, but the reader can easily imagine the results). After this analysis, summarising all information, we can induce as follows:

- In all images we can find two objects: 'Woman' and 'Vehicle'
- In some images, but not on all of them, there are also objects such as the 'Man'. Thus Men can be automatically considered as not important for the search criteria here
- Result: the computer finds and presents, as desired, all images with a Woman and a Vehicle, for example the images given in Fig. 2.3.

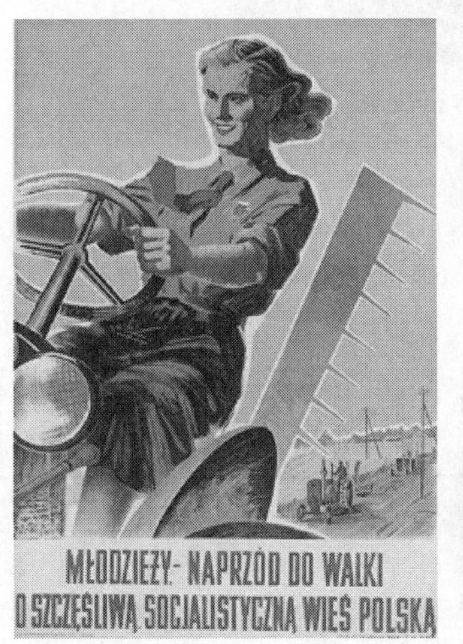

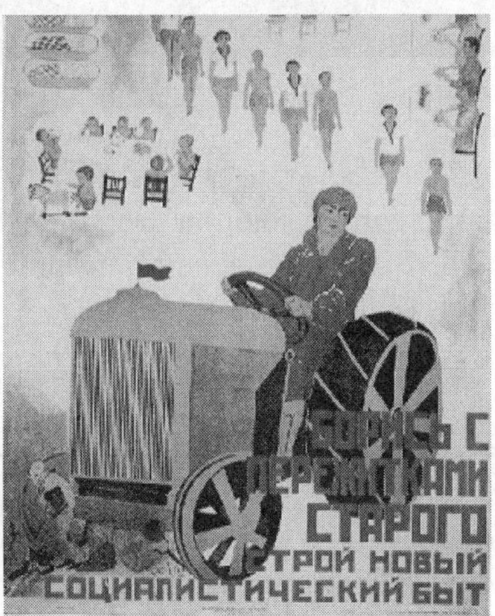

Fig. 2.3.a–b. Wrong images selected from the data base

(For people unfamiliar with ex-communist countries it is wise to comment on the actual joke at this point: the selected images are very well known allegories presented on Soviet posters labelled as 'all young girls ought to work on tractors').

It is very easy to find out that the method of image selection discovered by the automate is wrong in this situation; examples of correctly selected images from the data base are shown on Fig. 2.4.

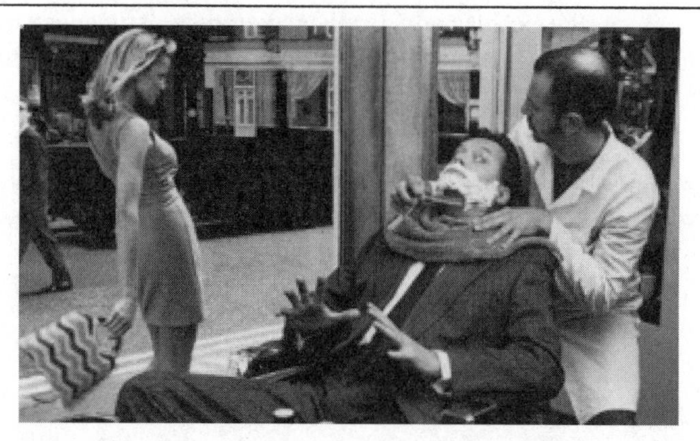

Fig. 2.4. A proper result of the semantic search process

This is the correct solution even though Fig. 2.4. does not contain 'Vehicle' at all. In fact the general meaning of all presented images is contained in this sentence:

Now we can see, why (and because of who) a man's life can often be so short!

Of course, this was only a joke (for which we apologise...). The issue itself, however, is quite serious because very often images seemingly very different hide in fact semantically identical contents and, vice versa, apparently very similar images can have a drastically different meaning.

2.2. What does image understanding mean?

The joke presented in the previous section shows, that we need a method to extract some kind of semantic contents that are present on the image (picture), but that are not obviously noticeably on it. This task can be difficult due to the fact that the gist is often hidden and needs a precise **understanding** of the image rather than its simple analysis, segmentation and even recognition. Based on the analyses of many unquestionably serious examples (medical images) we shall try to formulate the following three assumptions:

- The problem of a correct interpretation of many medical images cannot be solved by means of traditional image processing, image analysis or pattern recognition.
- The only way is to formulate a new paradigm of image interpretation and to develop a new method for its full automation, based on the application of artificial advanced intelligence tools.
- Automatic reasoning of image semantic contents, performed with the use of picture analysis is called image automatic understanding.

The fundamental features of medical image automatic understanding (according to our proposal) can be listed as follows:

- We try to imitate the natural method in which a medical doctor thinks: he/she needs to understand the disease before making a formal diagnosis and choosing the right treatment.
- First we make a linguistic description of the of the image contents, using a special kind of image description language (see Chapter 3 and 4). Owing to this idea we can describe every image without specifying any limited number of *a priori* described classes.
- The linguistic description of an image content constructed in this manner is the basis for an understanding image diagnosis or for indexing multimedia data bases (see Chapter 4 and 5).

A very important difference between all traditional methods of automatic image processing (or recognition) and the new paradigm for image understanding is that there is one directional scheme of the data flow in the traditional methods; there are two-directional interactions between signals (features) extracted from the image analysis and expectations resulting from the knowledge of image contents, as given by experts (physicians). Let us look at Fig. 2.5 on which we can see a traditional chart representing image processing for medical purposes.

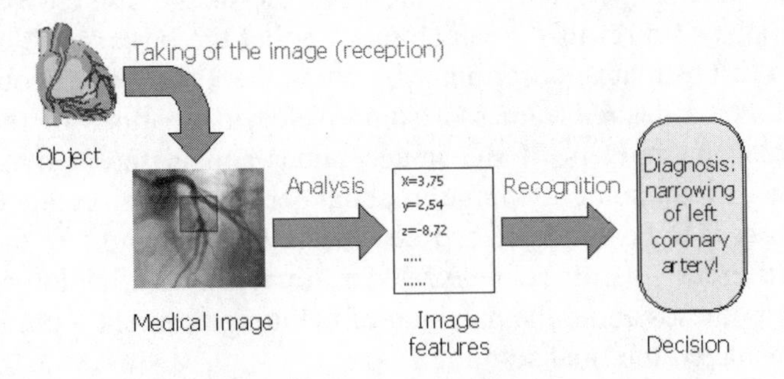

Fig. 2.5. Traditional method of medical image recognition

Unlike in this simple scheme representing classical recognition, in the course of image understanding we always have a **two-directional** flow of information (Fig. 2.6).

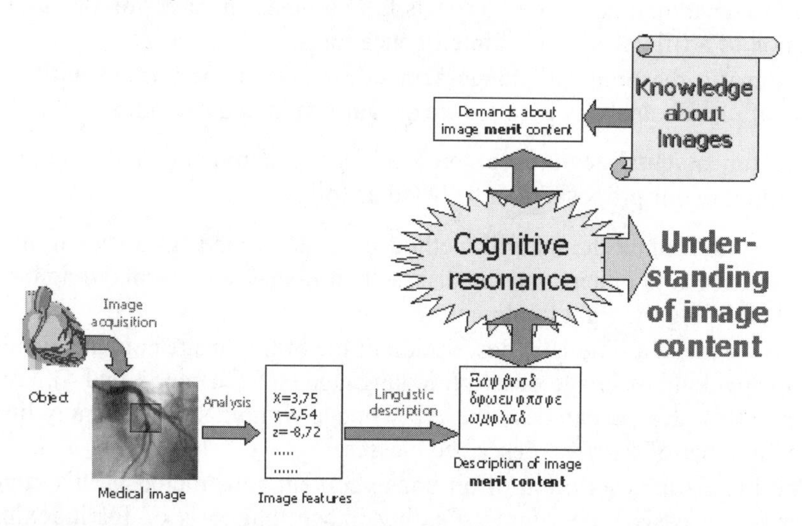

Fig. 2.6. The main paradigm of image understanding

On both figures presented above we can see that when we use the traditional pattern recognition paradigm, all processes of image analysis are based on a feed-forward scheme (one-directional flow of signals). On the contrary, when we apply automatic understanding of the image, the total input data stream (all features obtained as a result of an analysis of the image under consideration) must be compared with the stream of **demands** generated by a dedicated **source of knowledge**. The demands are always connected with a specific (selected) hypothesis of the image content semantic interpretation. As a result we can emphasise that the proposed 'demands' are a kind of postulates, describing (based on the knowledge about the image contents) the desired values of some (selected) features of the image. The selected parameters of the image under consideration must have desired values when some assumption about semantic interpretation of the image content is to be validated as true. When the parameters of the input image are different – it **can** be interpreted as a **partial** falsification of one of possible hypotheses about the meaning of the image content – but it still cannot be considered the final solution.

Due to this specific model of inference we labelled our mechanism the 'cognitive resonance'. This name is appropriate to our ideas because during the comparison process of features calculated for the input image and demands generated by the source of knowledge – we can observe an amplification of some hypotheses (about the meaning of the image content) while other (competitive) hypotheses weaken. It is very similar to the interferential image formed during a mutual activity of two wave sources: at some points in space waves can add to one another, in other points there are opposite phases and the final result is near zero.

Such structure of the system for image understanding corresponds to one of very well known models of natural visual perception by man, named 'knowledge based perception'. The human eye cannot recognise an object if the brain has no template for such likeness. This holds true even when the brain knows the object, but shown in another view, which means that other signals are coming to the visual cortex. People find it hard to believe how strong and how important this mechanism is in our own perception process. Still, this fact remains true. For example, let us try to recognise the face of a very well-known man presented on Fig 2.7.

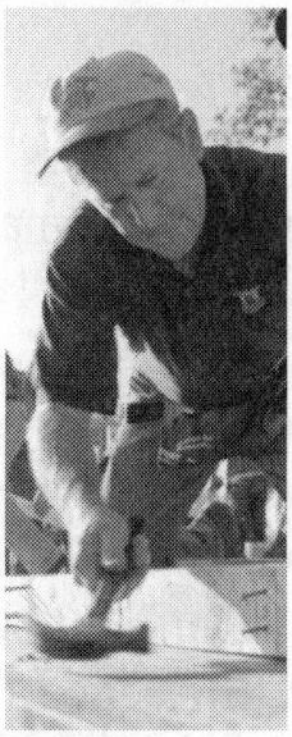

Fig. 2.7. Who is the man in the picture on the right?

If you want to do this experiment to get a proper result, you must try to recognise the face rather quickly. After a long time of thinking your brain can transform the image to a known form and you will find the solution. But at first sight it is not so easy, is it?

And please do not look at the next page, where in Fig. 2.8 you will find the correct solution immediately!

The right answer is of course ... President George W. Bush working on a Habitat for a Humanity house in Tampa, Tuesday, June 5, 2001. (Fig. 2.7 is an official WHITE HOUSE PHOTO by Eric Draper). The correct answer to the proposed quiz can be found in one second when you look at the same face but in a more familiar situation presented on Fig. 2.8.

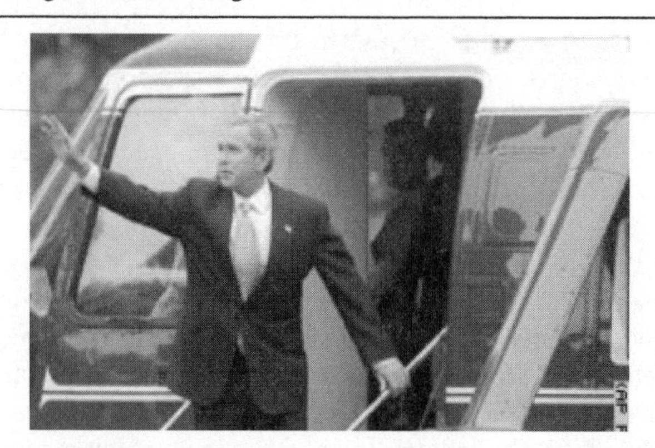

Fig. 2.8. This situation is easier because it is typical and known

The quiz above was our next joke (for which we apologise once again). Nevertheless it demonstrates a very general rule: during the observation process human brain generates hypotheses at every moment, based of its knowledge. Natural perception in fact is not just the processing of visual signals obtained by eyes. It is mainly a mental cognitive process, based on hypotheses generation and its real-time verification. The verification is performed by comparing permanently the selected features of an image with expectations taken from earlier visual experience.

Our method of image understanding is based on the same processes with a difference that it is performed by computers. Let us analyse such processes in more detail.

2.3. Linguistic description of images

A very important aspect of the automatic image understanding method described in this book is a very close connection between our whole methodology and mathematical linguistics, especially a linguistic description of images. There are two important reasons for the selection of linguistic (syntactic) methods of image description for the fundamental tool to understanding images.

The first one derives from the fact, that (as has already been mentioned) in the case of understanding we have no classes or templates known *a priori*. In fact the possible number of potential classes goes to infinity. So we must use a tool that offers us possibilities to describe a potentially infinite number of categories. This means that it is necessary to have a tool to **generate** descriptions of classes rather than to point to classes described *a pri-*

ori. For this the only suitable tool is a language that can generate an infinite number of sentences. Every mechanism generating a finite list of identifiers or names in this case is absolutely insufficient.

The second reason for using a linguistic approach to automatic image understanding is connected with the fact that in the linguistic approach, after processing, we obtain a description of the image content without the use of any classification known *a priori* due to the fact that even the criteria of the classification are constructed and developed during the automatic reasoning process. This is possible because of very a strong generalisation mechanism included into (or built in) the grammar parsing process. Owing to formal and powerful technologies for automatic parsing of all linguistic formulas (describing actual images), we can recommend the mathematical linguistic technology as the most powerful technology for any generalisation.

In fact, every grammar is always a tool for generalisation. When we write in a natural form 'dog', 'cat', 'tree', 'car', we describe actual objects. But after this we can use grammar and obtain a much more general category, 'noun', which is much more useful to understanding the roles of all objects under consideration and their mutual relationships.

The only problem is connected with a correct adjustment of the terms and methods of formal grammars and artificial languages to application in the field of images (e.g. languages for computer programming rather than strings of symbols, as it is in natural languages and even most artificial languages). The problem is very well known to specialists but, for the completeness of our presentation; let us explain some fundamental ideas. Readers familiar with syntactic approaches to image processing are requested skip the rest of this chapter.

When we try to build a language for the description of images we must start with fundamental definitions of elements belonging to the suitable graph grammar. Let us assume that we must build a grammar for the description of a class of landscapes, similar to images presented on Fig. 2.9.

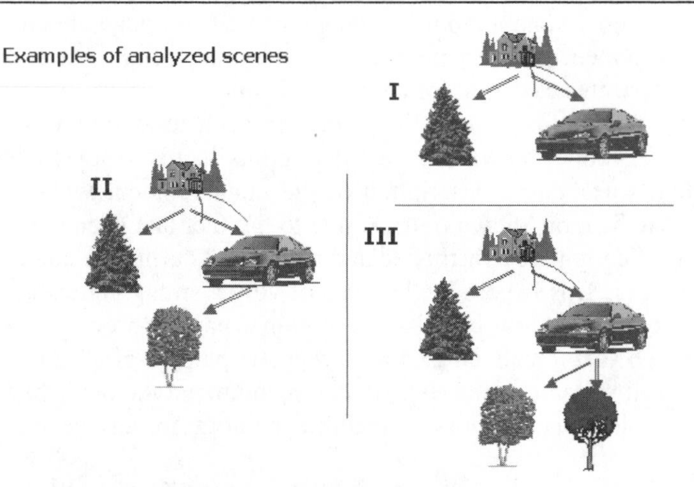

Fig. 2.9. Class of images for syntactic description

An analysis of the scenes under consideration shows that we have some classes of graphic objects ('primitives') which can be built into the grammar as substantives (nouns). We also have some classes of relations between objects, which can be treated as the verbs of our grammar. So the vocabulary of grammar for the images under consideration can be shown as on Fig. 2.10.

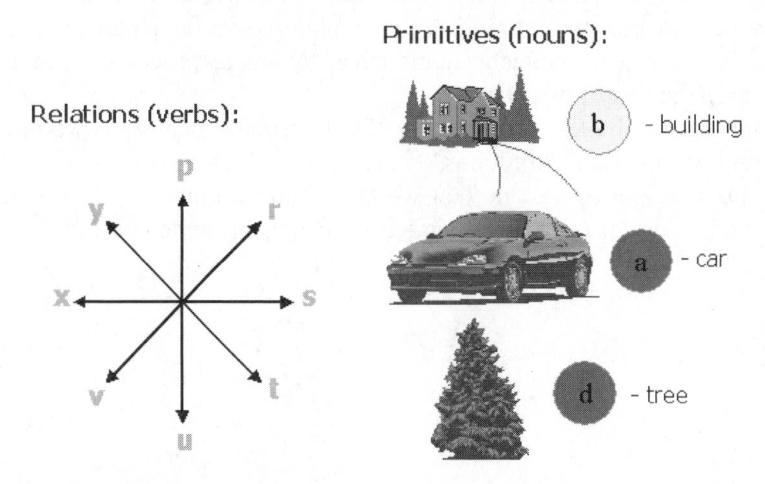

Fig. 2.10. Elements of vocabulary

Using the proposed vocabulary we can replace every landscape image with an equivalent scheme for the grammar, as shown on Fig. 2.11. (Please compare this figure with Fig. 2.9. for the analysis of source images and with Fig. 2.10. for considering grammar rules).

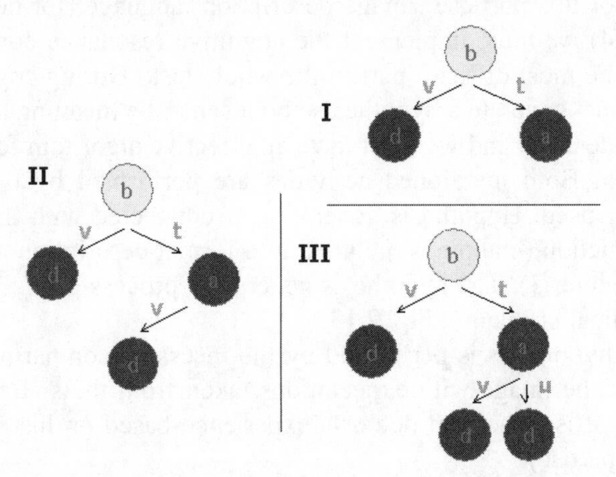

Fig. 2.11. Symbolic representation of the scene before describing it in terms of graph-grammar

On the basis of such symbolic description of the image under consideration we can also use symbolic notations for elements of vocabulary; for every image they obtain a representation in terms of terminal symbols belonging to the definition of the grammar used (see Fig. 2.12. and also Chapter 3).

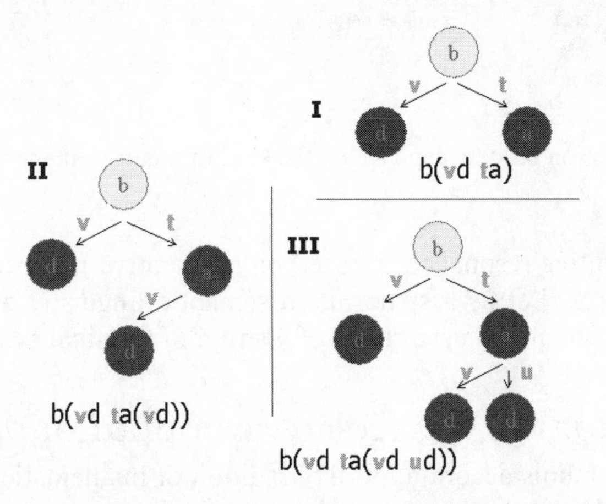

Fig. 2.12. Conversion of a graph diagram of the image into its symbolic description

2.4. The use of graph grammar to cognitive resonance

After a final description of the image-using elements of a selected (or, most typically, built for this purpose) image description language (for details refer to Chapter 4) we must implement the cognitive resonance concept. It is, of course, the most difficult part in the whole task. During cognitive resonance we must generate a hypothesis about semantic meaning of the image under consideration and we must have an effective algorithm for its on-line verification. Both mentioned activities are performed by the parser of the grammar used. Hypothesis generation is connected with the use of a selected production (mappings included into formal description of the grammar – see Chapter 3). The hypothesis generation process depends very much on the medical problem – Fig. 2.13.

Verification of the hypothesis is performed by the incessant comparing of selected features of the image with expectations taken from the source of knowledge (mostly it is a medical doctor's experience based on his or her previous visual expertise).

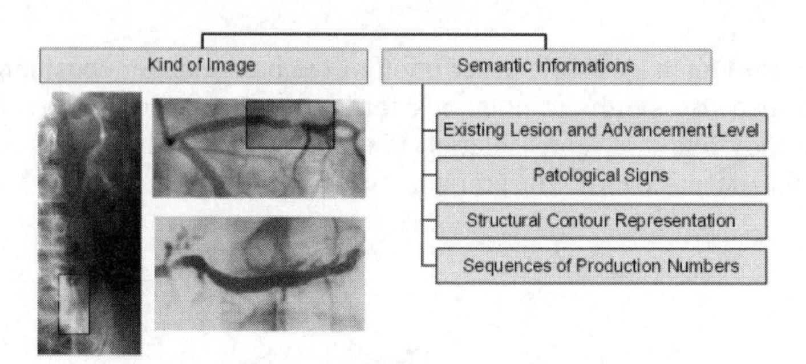

Fig. 2.13. Hypothesis generation process depends on the kind of medical image

The main idea of cognitive resonance is based on an iterative performance of the following steps. Let us assume that a semantic linguistic description of an image is done in the usual form of a string of terminal symbols:

$$\sigma\varepsilon\mu\alpha\nu\tau\psi\chi\zeta\nu\psi o\pi\iota\sigma\alpha\nu\alpha\lambda\iota\zeta o\omega\alpha\nu\varepsilon\gamma o o\beta\rho\alpha\zeta\upsilon\mu\alpha$$

We are using Greek symbols according to the tradition of mathematical linguistics and as a signal to show that a man does not need to understand symbols produced by the linguistic processor, it is enough if the parser can manage them.

Now the parsing process begins. Let us assume that the **working hypothesis number 1** about the meaning of this image leads to the assumption that the image must include at least one pattern:

οχζεκ

Parser starts the search process through all strings of terminal symbols describing (in terms of the used language) important semantic features of the analysed image.

The searching process fails, which means that strength of the working hypothesis no 1 is decreasing. Another working hypothesis leads to the assumption that the image must include at least one pattern:

χζνψ

This pattern can be found in the string:

σεμαντψχζνψοπισαναλιζοωανεγοοβραζυμα

which means that our working hypothesis no 2 can now be considered more probable. Yet we are still not quite sure whether the hypothesis is true or not because for its full validation it is necessary to test also other assumptions taken from this hypothesis and from all other hypotheses.

The description of cognitive resonance presented here is, of course, more simplified. In fact the set of methods and formulas used by the real parser designed by us especially for this work is a lot more complicated! That one will be shown in Chapter 4 on practical examples.

3. Formal Bases for the Semantic Approach to Medical Image Processing Leading to Image Understanding Technology

3.1 Fundamentals of syntactic pattern recognition methods

This chapter presents the basic terms of the formal language and finite state automata theory that are associated with syntactic pattern recognition methods. The symbols and terms introduced here will be used throughout this book; the formalisms introduced here will be used by the Authors in cognitive analyses of images presented in this book.

3.1.1 Definitions and basic formalisms associated with syntactic pattern recognition methods

Definition 1.1. Alphabet Σ is a finite set of symbols.

Definition 1.2. A word above alphabet Σ is every finite string of symbols composed of alphabet Σ symbols.

Definition 1.3. Vocabulary Σ^+ is a set of all meaningful[1] words above alphabet Σ.

[1] A word is regarded as 'meaningful' if it is employed during the use of the analysed language. In some cases vocabulary Σ^+ is identical with a set of all words above alphabet Σ. In such cases a simple combinatorial procedure is sufficient and any finite combination of symbols, with no exceptions, belonging to alphabet Σ belongs to vocabulary Σ^+. In languages applied in practice there is always

Definition 1.4. A word without any symbol is called an **empty word** and denoted by λ.

Definition 1.5. An extended vocabulary is set $\Sigma^*=\Sigma+\cup\lambda$

Definition 1.6. The number n of symbols in a word $w = x_1 \ldots x_n$ is called the length of the word 'w' and denoted by $|w|=n$ while $|\lambda|=0$.

Definition 1.7. **Attributive grammars**

Attributive grammar is defined as a quadruple $G=(V_n, V_t, SP, STS)$; where V_n, V_t are finite sets of non-terminal and terminal symbols, STS is the grammar start symbol and the SP is a production set of which each consists of two parts: a syntactic rule and a semantic rule.

The syntactic rules have the form of: $X\rightarrow a$, for $X\in V_n$ and $a \in V_n \cup V_t$

On the other hand, the semantic rules are given in the following form:

$$Y_1 = f_1(X_{11}, X_{12}, \ldots, X_{1n1}, Y_1, \ldots, Y_n), Y_2 = f_2(X_{21}, X_{22}, \ldots, X_{2n2}, Y_1, \ldots, Y_n), \ldots Y_n = f_n(X_{n1}, X_{n2}, \ldots, X_{n\,nn}, Y_1, \ldots, Y_n)$$

where X_{ij} $(1\leq i\leq n,\ 1\leq j\leq n_i)$ are attributes of terminal or non-terminal symbols, f_i $((1\leq i\leq n)$ are the assigned functions or appropriately defined semantic procedures; Y_i $((1\leq i\leq n)$ are attributes or defined variables employed in semantic actions.

Definition 1.8. A context-free grammar is a grammar whose productions have the form:

$A \rightarrow \gamma$, where $A\in\Sigma_N$, $\gamma\in\Sigma^+$

i.e. a non-terminal A is replaced by a non-empty γ sequence made of any combination of terminal and non-terminal symbols.

The notation $\eta\rightarrow\gamma$ denotes *a direct derivation step* in grammar G. In other words if η and γ have the respective forms of $\eta=\sigma_1\chi\sigma_2$ and $\gamma=\sigma_1\tau\sigma_2$ (for both contexts σ_1, σ_2), then there exists a production $\chi\rightarrow\tau\in P$.

The notation $\eta \xrightarrow{*} \gamma$ denotes an *indirect* derivation in grammar G. This means that there exists a sequence:

$\eta_0, \eta_1 \ldots \eta_k$ such that $\eta_0 = \eta$, $\eta_k = \gamma$ and $\eta_i\rightarrow\eta_{i+1} \in P$ (are direct derivation steps).

---

a certain ***redundancy***, i.e. only some symbol strings carry meaning while most other symbol strings (that can be built) from alphabet Σ have no meaning.

Definition 1.9. **Language** generated by grammar G is the set:

$L(G) = \{\gamma : \gamma \in \Sigma_T^* \text{ such that } S \xrightarrow{*} \gamma\}$

or the set of all terminal words that may be derived from the S grammar start symbol.

Definition 1.10. A context-free grammar G=(V_N, V_T, SP, STS) is the LR(k)-type grammar (for k≥0) if, for each derivation step of forms:

$STS \Rightarrow^R \mu A\omega \Rightarrow \mu\chi\omega,\ \mu\in V^*,\ \omega\in V_T^*,\ A\rightarrow\chi\in SP$

$STS \Rightarrow^R \mu' B\omega' \Rightarrow \mu'\gamma\omega',\ \mu'\in V^*,\ \omega'\in V_T^*,\ B\rightarrow\gamma\in SP$

The condition $(|\mu\chi|+k): \mu\chi\omega = (|\mu'\gamma|+k): \mu'\gamma\omega'$ implies that : $\mu=\mu'$, A=B, $\chi=\gamma$

where: $\Rightarrow^R$ denotes the right-hand derivation (right-hand derivation or a derivation step) in grammar, i.e. in each new step a new text string is derived from the rightmost non-terminal symbol.

$V=V_T\cup V_N$, $V^*=\{\mu: \mu=x_1x_2...x_n,\ n\geq 1,\ x_i\in V \text{ for } i=1...n\}\cup\lambda$ (λ is an empty symbol)

$V_T^*=\{\omega: \omega=y_1y_2...y_m,\ m\geq 1,\ y_i\in V_T \text{ for } i=1...m\}\cup\lambda$,

$$k:w=\begin{cases} w, & when\ |w|<k \\ \alpha, & when\ \omega=\alpha\gamma\ and\ |\alpha|=k \end{cases}$$

Due to the fact that in the class of context-free grammars, apart from a wide sub-group of LR(k)-type grammars, also a sub-class of LL(k) grammars is differentiated that are widely used in practical syntactic analysis tasks to make the picture complete, we shall give also a definition of this grammar class.

Definition 1.11. A context-free grammar G=(V_N, V_T, SP, STS) is a LL(k)-type grammar for a given k ≥ 0 if for any derivation:

$STS\ {}^*\!\!\Rightarrow^L \gamma_1 A\gamma_2 \Rightarrow \gamma_1\sigma\gamma_2\ {}^*\!\!\Rightarrow^L \gamma_1\eta_1,\qquad \gamma_1, \eta_1\in V_T^*,\ \sigma, \gamma_2\in V^*,\ A\in V_N$

$STS\ {}^*\!\!\Rightarrow^L \gamma_1 A\gamma_2 \Rightarrow \gamma_1\tau\gamma_2\ {}^*\!\!\Rightarrow^L \gamma_1\eta_2,\qquad \eta_1\in V_T^*,\ \tau\in V^*$

The condition ($k:\eta_1 = k:\eta_2$) implies that : $\underline{\sigma=\tau}$

where: $\Rightarrow^L$ denotes the left-hand derivation (left-hand derivation or a derivation step) in a grammar, i.e. at every step the text string is derived from the leftmost non-terminal symbol.

A feature of these grammars is that there are deterministic syntactic analysers for them (automata with a stack) recognising languages generated by such grammars. An LL(k)-type automaton works in the following way: it scans the input sequence from left to right reading its subsequent elements (letter L in LL) and at the output it generates a figure sequence of the left-hand derivation production for the input sequence (the second letter L in LL). These automata are stack generation-type ones, performing the so-called top-down analysis and examining no more than *k* input symbol at any one step. The top-down analysis is based on a derivation of the analysed input sequence at the stack top, beginning with the grammar start symbol.

However, due to that the reduction-type analysis is more general than the generation one, in practical applications reduction parsers are used more frequently. Such analysers are constructed in order to analyse language elements generated by LR(k)-type grammars. An additional advantage of this type of analysers is that they detect syntactic errors as quickly as possible, that is immediately after at the input appears a symbol indicating that the generated sequence does not belong to the language generated by the grammar introduced. It is for these reasons as well as due to the fact resulting from theorem 1.1, i.e. that each LL(k)-type grammar is simultaneously a LR(k)-type grammar (the reverse inclusion does not hold true), further considerations will be limited only to LR(k)-type grammars.

THEOREM 1.1 Each LL(k) grammar is also a LR(k) grammar [65]
No proof

Definition 1.12. An LR(1)-class automaton (or LR(1) automaton for grammar G is the sequence:

LRA(G)=(Q, V_n,V_t, SP, q_0,*next*, *reduce*)

where: Q is a finite nonempty set of automaton states, V_n, V_t are finite sets of non-terminal and terminal symbols, Sp is a production set, $q_0 \in Q$ is the initial automaton state.

The function of the next state, *next,* is determined as:

$$next\colon Q \times (V_n \cup V_t \cup \{\$\})^* \rightarrow Q \cup \{stop\}$$

and satisfies the following conditions (symbol $ is a limiter of the input sequence):
1. *next*(q, λ)=q
2. *next*(q, αx)=next(next(q, α), x)

The reduction function *reduce* is determined as:

$$reduce: Q \times (V_n \cup V_t \cup \{\$\})^* \to 2^{SP}$$

On the other hand, the LR(1) automaton works in the following way: it scans (analyses) the input sequence from left to right reading its subsequent elements (hence the letter L in LR). At the output it generates the inverse of the right-hand derivation of the input sequence (letter R in LR), processing no more that 1 input symbol in each step.

LR(1)-type automata belong to the group of reduction analysers, controlled by means of the so-called parser steering table. In practical terms this means that LR(1)-class parsers are implemented in the software with the use of a state table and by means of numbers of the reduction productions. The automaton operation is determined by two functions describing the analyser current state and defined in order to carry out a complete reduction analysis. These functions are: *action procedure* and *goto*.

The syntactic analysis is started from the initial automaton configuration, i.e. the application of the *action procedure* defined for the q_0 initial state and the first input sequence symbol.

The types of actions defined for the syntax analyser while the analysis is being conducted have been presented in Table 3.1

Table 3.1. Actions performed by syntax analyser during the input sequence analysis

Action	Meaning
Shift	The first symbol from the input is shifted to the stack top
Reduce	The right-hand side of one of productions is on the stack top and as a result of a reduction it is replaced with the left-hand side of this production
Error	State of error and discontinuation of further analysis. The input sequence has not been correctly defined by means of grammar derivation rules
Accept	Approval of the input sequence as a correctly recognised and completed analysis.

In order to describe the functioning of *action procedure* and *goto* functions, the notion of LR(1)-type automaton configuration will be introduced:

Definition 1.13. The configuration of LR(1) automaton is a triple:

$$(stack,\ input,\ output)$$

where: stack $\in(V_n \cup V_t \cup Q)^*$ contains a sequence composed of terminal symbols, non-terminal symbols and automaton states (the rightmost symbol determines the stack top); the *input* $\in\Sigma^*\$$ is defined by a sequence of terminal symbols at the automaton input, ended with $, the symbol of the input sequence end (the leftmost symbol is the first symbol in this sequence); the *output* contains a sequence of production numbers used for reduction so far during the input word (sequence) analysis so far.

For the syntactic analyser the transfer function is given in the form of a steering table (the methods governing the construction of such tables can be found in [65]) and determined with the use of the *action procedures* and the *goto* function defined as follows:

action procedure: $Q \times (V_t \cup \{\$\}) \rightarrow Q \cup SP \cup \{accept, error\}$

This procedure executes two types of actions (provided in Table 3.1.):

a) *shift* when the *action procedure* $(q_n,a)=q_m$, $q_m \in Q$ and the automaton configuration changes in the following way (as described in Table 3.2):

Table 3.2. Changes in the LR(1) automaton configurations during the 'shift action

Stack	Input	Output
	initial configuration (in the state q_0)	
$\ldots q_n$	$\leftarrow ab\ldots$	–
	Configuration in the subsequent step (i.e. after the shift action)	
$\ldots q_n a q_m$	$b\ldots$	–

b) *reduce* when *action procedure* $(q_n,a)=p_i$; where $p_i \in SP$ denotes a production having the number *i* and form $p_i:A \to \beta$ whose the right-hand side (handle) has length *k* (i.e. $|\beta|=k$) and the form $\beta=x_{n-k}...x_n$; and on top of the stack there is the same handle (whose symbols might be separated by symbols of automaton states). In such a case the reduction can be applied while the topmost stack handle is replaced by the left-hand production side (reduction analysis) whose handle (i.e. the right side) in on the stack. The number of the production applied is written at the automaton output.

Due to that after the reduction, at the stack top there is a non-terminal of a left-hand production side with *i*-th number, rather than the automaton state symbol, it is necessary to perform the *goto* action specified in the following way:

$$goto\colon\ Q \times V_n \to Q \cup \{error\}$$

This function causes the automaton to move to the new state whose symbol appears at the top of the stack.

As a result of execution of the *reduce* action and the function *goto* following it, the automaton configuration changes in a manner shown in Table 3.3 (bold letters indicate the production handle of the stack top).

Table 3.3. Changes of LR(1) automaton configuration during the execution of the '*reduce*' and '*goto*' actions

Stack	Input	output
Original configuration (in state q_n) On the stack top the handle of the production $p_i:A\to\beta$ $(=x_{n-k}...x_n)$ is visible		
$...x_{n-k-1}q_{n-k-1}\mathbf{x_{n-k}q_{n-k}...x_nq_n}$	ab...	-
Configuration in the subsequent step, i.e. after action reduces (state q_{n-k-1}). The handle reduced to the left-hand production side, that is to A. Production number written at the output		
$...\ x_{n-k-1}q_{n-k-1}A$	ab...	i
Performing the goto function for the topmost state and non-terminal and transition to a new state. $goto(q_{n-k-1},A)=q_m$		
$...\ x_{n-k-1}q_{n-k-1}Aq_m$	ab...	i

Definition 1.14. A multiple-input sequential transducer is a quintuple defined in the following way [56]:

$$ST=(Q, \Sigma_T, \Delta, \delta, Q_0)$$

Where: Q – finite set of states, Σ_T – finite set of input symbols (terminals), Δ – finite set of output symbols, $Q_0 \subset Q$ – set of initial states, δ – transition function defined as: δ: $Q x \Sigma^*_T \longrightarrow Q x \Delta^*$.

The notation $\delta(q,\gamma)=(q,\eta)$ means that after reading the input sequence $\gamma \in \Sigma^*T$, the transducer moves from state q to q' and writes at the output sequence $\eta \in \Delta^*$. For the input sequence of $\gamma \in \Sigma^*T$ terminal symbols, the sequence $\eta=ST(\gamma)$ is the output text string from the transducer if and only if there are the following the sequences:

$$\gamma_1,...,\gamma_k \in \Sigma^*{}_T\ ,\ \eta_1,...,\eta_k \in \Delta^*\ ,\ q_1,...,q_k \in Q$$

Satisfying the following conditions:

1. $\gamma = \gamma_1,...,\gamma_k$,
2. $\eta = \eta_1,...,\eta_k$,
3. $\delta(q_i,\gamma_{i+1}) = (q_{i+1},\eta_{i+1})$ for i=0, 1,..., k-1, $q_0 \in Q_0$.

An analysis with the use of sequential transducers is extremely effective when a description of the looked-for lesions is introduced in the form of languages describing shape features. This is especially important in diagnosing structures particularly complex in their morphology. In further sections of this book an approach using such languages as an additional tool describing and analysing the pancreatic ducts will be presented.

Definition 1.15. Expansive G_{edt} tree grammar generating trees with directed and labelled edge, i.e. EDT trees. It is defined as a set of five other sets defined as follows [56]:

$$G_{edt}=(\Sigma, \Gamma, r, P, Z)$$

where Σ is a set of terminal and non-terminal vertex labels, *r* is a function assigning to the tree vertex the number of its successors (children), *Z* is finite set of start trees, Γ is a set of edge labels and *P* is a production set with the following form:

$$A \rightarrow a(\tau_1 A_1\ \tau_2 A_2 ...\ \tau_{r(a)} A_{r(a)})$$

where: A_1, $A_2 ... A_{r(a)}$ are non-terminal vertexes while 'a' is a terminal vertex; $\tau_1,\tau_2 ... \tau_{r(a)}$ are edge labels.

The right-hand side of the production $a(\tau_1 A_1, \tau_2 A_2 .....\tau_{r(a)} A_{r(a)})$ denotes an EDT tree written in the parentheses form. The tree has a root and r(a) successor leafs designated labelled A_1, A_2.... $A_{r(a)}$, connected to the root by means of r(a) edges labelled as a τ_1, τ_2.....$\tau_{r(a)}$ respectively and directed from the root to the leaves.

The formalism of tree grammars defined in this way will be used later in the book for analysis of renal pelvis morphology.

3.1.2 Principles of syntax analysers operation

The group of most common compilers of syntax analysers includes the YACC compiler developed by the AT&T concern as well as the Bison software of the Free Software Foundation Inc, [16]. These software pieces are general-purpose compilers creating syntax analysers capable of simple syntactic analysis in image perception systems. Such analysers are generated by them based on a formal notation of a grammar belonging to the Look-Ahead-LR(1) class of context-free grammars and they take on the form of source code of the C programming language.

In order to perform a syntactic analysis (parsing) of language expressions, it is required that they be first described with a context-free grammar generating a given formal language. Such a language might generate recurrent productions but at least one of them must be a recurrence-free production. Unfortunately, due to difficulties and the complexity of the automation parser steering tables generation process, not all types of context-free grammars can be compiled by YACC and Bison analysers. The range of input grammars is narrowed down to a smaller group of LALR(1)-type grammars. Such grammars are characterised by that it is possible to make an unequivocal syntactic analysis of the input sequence viewing only at one token (symbol) from the automaton input.

In formal grammar description each element describing the input units or syntactic sets is called 'a symbol', as in definitions quoted in previous sections. Symbols produced through a grouping of several smaller symbols, in accordance with grammar rules, are called 'non-terminal symbols'. Those that cannot be further divided are called 'terminal' symbols and in the case of syntax analyser software implementation, they are referred to as '**tokens**'.

If we use the example of C programming language, the tokens (grammar terminal symbols) can be identifiers, constants, key words, arithmetic operators, etc. Non-terminal symbols on the other hand can describe for example expressions, declarations and definitions of functions. In our case that is in diagnosing various disease symptoms in the analysis of selected anatomic structures the tokens will be the smallest, indivisible elements describing the sought-for symptoms that is sections approximating them over the obtained width profiles. Non-terminal symbols define the major looked-for disease symptoms and any and all intermediate elements necessary to group terminal symbols in such a way that they describe the looked-for lesion.

One of elements from the set of non-terminal symbols is a distinguished element from which the generation of the whole language defined by an appropriate grammar begins. This element is called the start symbol, sometimes colloquially referred to as 'the grammar head'.

Parsers generated by the described generators read a sequence of tokens at the input; in subsequent steps they group them by means of reducing the stack topmost symbols, representing the right-hand side of one of productions, and by replacing them with the production left-hand side. If therefore the initial terminal symbol sequence is a sequence written in accordance with syntactic rules of a defined grammar, the reduction analysis outcome will be reduced by degrees to the initial grammar start symbol. If, however, the sequence does not belong to the language generated by the grammar, then during the analysis we shall receive information about a recognition error.

Apart from the syntax analysis of the input sequence, the generated syntax analysers are capable of performing semantic actions ascribed to individual productions. This one allows generating certain values or information being the result of the performed syntactic analysis. In the YACC and Bison compilers, semantic actions are written together with individual productions by means of language C programming instructions. Every time the parser uses for reduction one of productions, simultaneously it performs a semantic action assigned to it. Usually the objective of such actions is to compute the semantic value of the whole input sequence (expression) on the basis of semantic values of this expression's individual components.

Let us imagine, for example, a rule which sets forth the value of one given expression as the sum of values of two other sub-expressions. At the moment the analyser recognises this expression and attempts to compute its value (with the use of a semantic action), each of the component values (i.e. the values of sub-expressions) will be already known. This will allow it simply to add them and to calculate the required, superior expression.

In the analysis of medical images, semantic actions of some productions will be aimed also to determine the numerical values specifying the height and length of the diagnosed pathology, on the width diagram. These parameters will be then used as additional information useful in diagnosing ambiguous or dubious cases or symptoms.

The result of YACC and Bison software operation, receiving grammar description at the input, are parser procedures for these grammars written in the source code of the C programming language.

These parsers, placed in the main software piece and after compilation, perform a reduction analysis of expressions given at the input and they recognise whether they are compliant with rule of the introduced grammar. In the course of the analysis, the parser reads subsequent tokens from the input, calling the *lex analyser* procedure, defined precisely for this purpose by its developer.

The main procedure of the syntax analyser is the implementation of the parser steering table for the defined grammar. Another procedure, crucial for a correct analysis and necessary for the author to define the grammar, is the error-handling procedure. The latter informs about errors encountered during the analysis.

The general structure of the input file, together with a notation of the analysed grammar for YACC and Bison software pieces, is as follows:

```
%{
declaration of the C language
%}
software declarations
%%
grammar rules
%%
additional language C instructions
```

The symbols '%%', '%}, {%' are separation symbols. They separate individual sections in the file with the grammar notation.

In the section of language C declarations there can be defined types and variables employed in semantic actions. Besides, pre-processor commands can be used to define the macros and directives *#include,* to include heading sets.

In the YACC or Bison software declaration section, there are the declared names of terminal and non-terminal symbols, precedence operators and types of semantic values data.

Grammar rules define the method of construction of every non-terminal symbol from smaller elements, in particular from terminal symbols.

In additional language C instructions there can be any other additional instructions or procedures. However, usually this is the place where there is a defined procedure of the *yylex* lexical analysis and semantic procedures called in semantic actions for individual productions [16].

Parser algorithm operation

In syntactic analysis with the use of context-free grammars, the parsing algorithm is based on the operation automaton with a stack. The parser reads subsequent tokens from the input and places them on the top of the parser stack together with their corresponding semantic variables values. The operation of placing subsequent input symbols at the stack is called as the '*shift* operation'. When, at the stack top a group of several recently-read tokens (terminal symbols) makes the so-called handle, that is the right-hand side of one of productions, the parser can perform the reduction operation (*reduce)* grouping all these elements and replacing them, at the stack top, with a single non-terminal symbol from the left-hand side of this production. Simultaneously to the reduce operation, a semantic action defined for this production is also performed.

Semantic actions are usually interpreted as some values stored in global variables, corresponding to actual tokens appearing at the analyser input. The operational mode of such an analyser enforces usually the use of a 'union' data form to represent various data formats. Such data can take various forms, beginning with simple markers (flags), numerical data, through extended records, to addresses of more refined semantic procedures which can determine more advanced indicators (ratios) or launch complex rules, i.e. forming conclusions and allowing one to make initial diagnosis proposals. Of course, among the functional indicators there can also be addresses of procedures enhancing the analysis process, e.g. narrowing down the domain of subsequent input data or additional error correction mechanisms or restarting structural analysis. It is worth noticing that it is the semantic analysis that plays a key role in computer-aided understanding of semantic image contents. Apart from the knowledge and expectations defined by grammatical rules and the productions introduced, it is these very semantic actions that allow one to compute the morphometric parameters of the analysed lesions to be computed. Owing to the use of additional knowledge on the form, their location in a given organ, the advancement stage or even data about the pathogenic patient character, it is possible to reason these procedures more deeply, in order to move towards the meaning perception and drawing conclusions about the significance of the case analysed.

Let us come back to parser functioning. Its whole operating process is aimed to reduce (as a result of the *shift* and *reduce* functions) the whole token input sequence to a single non-terminal symbol, i.e. the grammar start symbol. Due to their operating method, this type of parsers is referred to as reduction parsers ('bottom-up parsers').

Another broad class of syntax analysers are the so-called generating parsers constructed for example for LL(1) context-free grammars. These parsers, however, are less universal and as a result less frequently used. Detailed information about this class of grammars and parsers can be found in [56].

As it has already been mentioned, the analysers considered in this section belong not only to the group of LR(1)-type parsers but also to a narrower grammar analysers subclass of the LALR(1)-type (look-ahead LR(1)). This results from that this type of analysers do not always reduce immediately at the time when at the stack top there is the right-hand side of one productions, but they 'view' (analyse) what is the next symbol at the input. Only then do they perform a further operation. This strategy is necessary for a correct syntactic analysis of many useful language sequences occurring in the majority of programming languages.

When a subsequent token appears at the input, it is not shifted to the top of the stack immediately but first it becomes a token to be viewed by the parser. In this situation the parser can first execute one or more *reduce* operations at the stack top before it makes the *shift* action on that element. It does not mean, however, that the parser performs all possible reductions that can be performed on stack top elements. Depending on the type of the token viewed, a delay in the application of several rules can be introduced. This situation occurs, for example, when the so-called *shift/reduce* conflict arises (the parser can either reduce the stack topmost expression or shift the next token from the input to the top of the stack. A classical example illustrating such a situation, showing also inability to avoid such states, is a syntactic analysis of two syntactically similar conditional instructions present in nearly all programming languages. These instructions are the following couple:

1. **if** (condition) **then** instruction
2. **if** (condition) **then** instruction **else** instruction

Assuming that **if, then** and **else** are terminal symbols recognised by the analyser as subsequent tokens, then in the case of analysis of a nested conditional instruction, for example such as:

if (condition) **then**
    if (condition) **then** instruction
    else instruction

at the moment the token **else** appears at the analyser input, the analyser can reduce the stack topmost expression (i.e. internal instruction **if**) through the application of the first rule; or it can shift the **else** token (perform the *shift* operation) to the top of the stack assuming that it will be followed by correctly defined further instructions which can be reduced using the second rule.

If there are *shift/reduce* conflicts, the discussed compilers solve them using as a standard the *shift* operation unless grammar authors change it by means of application of appropriate precedence operators. This property is often utilised by programmers writing their software in Pascal or C languages, there the use of nested conditional instructions from which has the **else** clause, is part of the most deeply nested instruction *if*. However, if in conflict situations the parser selected the *reduce* action, in a natural way this would result in that the **else** clause would correspond to the most external **if** instruction. Obviously, interpretation liberty can be obtained by means of application of operators (or key words) denoting the beginning and the end of complex instructions.

Such conflicts occur always when the introduced grammar is ambiguous. In order to prevent the parser generation, the adopted standard solution in such situations is to make the *shift* action. In the above-described example it results in belonging of part of **else** to the most internal *if* instruction. The compilers considered in this book notify every time when such conflicts arise.

Another kind of conflict are the *reduce/reduce* conflicts occurring in situations in which two or more grammar productions can be applied to reduce the stack topmost expression. Such situation usually means a serious grammatical error and it can lead to a malfunctioning of the generated parser.

In the course of analysis, generators handle such problems by selecting the grammar production that occurred earlier. We should note, however, that it is only as a temporary solution, rather than an optimal one. This means that the grammar author ought to analyse carefully this type conflicts and modify the grammar to remove them.

3.2 Characteristic features and advantages of structural approaches to medical image semantic analysis

In order to efficiently perform a task for the semantic interpretation of selected medical images, it is necessary to go through a number of stages leading to the semantic recognition with the application of image analysis syntactic methods. These stages are the implementation of a general philosophy underlying the application of syntactic methods, based in particular on the following:

1. Defining the primary components of the images analysed. Such components are the smallest, indivisible elements that can be separated in the original image as a result of its decomposition into smaller elements or sub-images. The primary components introduced allow one to introduce fully a syntactic description of the analysed structures. A set of words constituting such descriptions is then treated as a formal language.
2. Defining grammars of an appropriate class: for example, context-free and graph ones or shape features description languages; by means of the syntactic rules introduced they allow one to generate a previously-defined language.
3. Construction and implementation of analysing automata (syntactic parsers) which constitute the right recognising procedure and which allow one to detect the sought-for lesions by means of specifying whether the analysed automaton input sequence is an element generated by a given language grammar or not.

The extraordinary scarcity of literature on the subject discussing these issues and relating to applications of syntactic methods in the analysis of biomedical images results from some difficulties encountered by prospective authors of analysing systems based on these methods. Among their multitude especially two aspects are worth noticing. The first one is a need to make the recognition task with the use of syntactic analysis algorithms independent of the orientation and position of the analysed structure within the image. A great variety of shapes of individual cases that can occur in many tasks of anatomy structure morphology analysis as well as also a great variety of possible positions or orientations or location a given organ in relation to the structures result in that attempts at effective assessment of the morphology state with the use of computer software are extremely difficult or sometimes even impossible. The latter is due to the excessive number of possible cases that would have to be considered to make an unambiguous evaluation of the state of the examined structure.

Another major difficulty to overcome is a need to define a sufficiently strong lexical apparatus (i.e. a grammar formed) so that it belongs to one of grammar classes, for example a LR-type context-free grammar, where there are automatic parser generators. Unfortunately, not all grammar types have this property: not always do such deterministic syntax analysers exist which enable a recognition of the looked-for lesions in a clear and fully deterministic way. In the situation of a great variety of changes of the recognised structures, to recognise them correctly it can be required to define a very extensive grammar (extensive with regards to the number of introduced productions). This could mean a need to go beyond the class to which a grammar ought to belong, or it can mean the appearance of a grammar with conflicts. The desire to avoid such problems can lead to attempts of application of grammars with greater generative capacity, for example, context or phrase-structure grammars [56]. In their cases however, there can be problems with the construction of deterministic syntax analysers.

Fundamental differences between syntactic methods and well-known and widely applied methods, included into the group of minimal distance methods [52] which are successfully and willingly used for tasks such as recognition of hand-written and printed symbols, fingerprints, face features, satellite and oceanographic photographs, bio-potential patterns, etc., can be considered to be the major reasons hampering the achievement of even modest results in medical image cognitive analysis. An additional difficulty is frequent lack of existence of an ideal pattern. Thus the situation requires that an analysis of the examined medical images and diagnosis of selected diseases be conducted in a more general and flexible manner. The best illustrating example of such an analysis are applications described in the further sections. To diagnose pathological lesions in the morphology of these organs one cannot determine a full and finite didactic set, which would include all possible forms of pathologies listed. This is an obvious consequence of the fact that every patient is unique due to the occurrence of idiosyncratic anatomy differences. It is not possible therefore to provide a universal pattern in the form of one X-ray or MRI photograph specifying a model or standard shape of a healthy organ. As it has already been said there are idiosyncratic differences of organ shapes ensuing from the patient's age, sex, race, etc. All these result in that such cases classical image recognition methods are insufficient to conduct a holistic analysis whose result is a complete diagnosis of the looked-for disease symptoms.

Due to the fact that in medical image analysis there are difficulties with supplying a representative and at the same time a universal model, it is not possible to use, on the exclusivity basis, algorithms and computer-aided learning methods. Nor is it possible to apply measurement methods of the similarity or differentiation of the examined images in order to analyse these structure in an unequivocal manner. This means that in this case it is necessary to use such intelligent image recognition methods, which not only enable to process and detect simple objects, but also enable a wider semantic analysis and determination of features of extremely complex structures.

Lack of research (conducted at a wide scale) on the application of syntactic analysis methods of medical images, related to the previously listed difficulties, resulted in the appearance of a certain methodology and application gap found in scientific research conducted by many scientific research centres. This is connected with diagnosing many diseases which have symptoms seen in the form of organ morphological lesions and in works connected with development of computer systems supporting medical diagnosis.

It is worthwhile to emphasise at this point the great importance of these issues, in particular the scientific and application values associated with their use for cognitive analysis of medical images.

Owing to the developed methodology, the approach to analysis of selected medical images presented further in the book will be holistic. It will develop a cross-section through the most important operations and stages leading from the first actions of initial improvement of the examined images to the final recognition of the looked-for lesions.

It is also worth mentioning that the methods of syntactic medical image description presented in further sections constitute an attempt at automation of a human-specific process of medical meaning understanding of a given organ shape on a digital image and that they are not just an attempt at simple recognition (i.e. qualification into a pre-defined class). This is therefore an attempt at perceiving, that is a deeper understanding of the examined image [60].

A diagnosis can result from such automatic shape understanding; it is also possible to draw many other medical conclusions from it, too. Such information can relate to a method of treatment, for example: depending on the shape and locations of pathological lesions described in the grammar, different therapies can be recommended:

- conservative (with the use of pharmacological or physiotherapy means, for example: a massage or diathermy).
- Acting by means of remotely operating physical agents, for example destroying neoplasms with ionising beams of radiation or lithotrypsis taking advantage of ultrasounds: low-invasive treatment of artery dilation with aortal tubes.
- Treatment executed with the use of laparoscope techniques
- Treatment on an open operation field, divided into operations of organ complete removal and organ partial resections.

Another type of important diagnostic information is the looked-for correlation between the pathological form of an organ lesion described by the grammar and the treatment outcome known (ex-post). Based on this one can formulate, for new cases of the hypothesis appearing later, forecasts of the patient's future state.

4. Examples of Structural Pattern Analysis and Medical Image Understanding Application to Medical Diagnosis

4.1. Introduction

This chapter will present the results of actual medical applications of the new approach described in previous chapters. We shall try to demonstrate that the structural pattern analysis can be regarded as an effective tool for medical image understanding, replacing simple recognition (Figure 4.1). Structural image analysis can be considered as a totally new approach to the analysis and description of shapes of selected organs in medical imaging in general. Examples of syntactic methods of pattern recognition application for the understanding and analysis of selected medical images presented in this chapter show their usefulness for early diagnosis of some diseases of selected organs. Analysis results of investigations based on structural analysis of selected types of medical images confirm very good properties of the proposed methodology and algorithms under consideration.

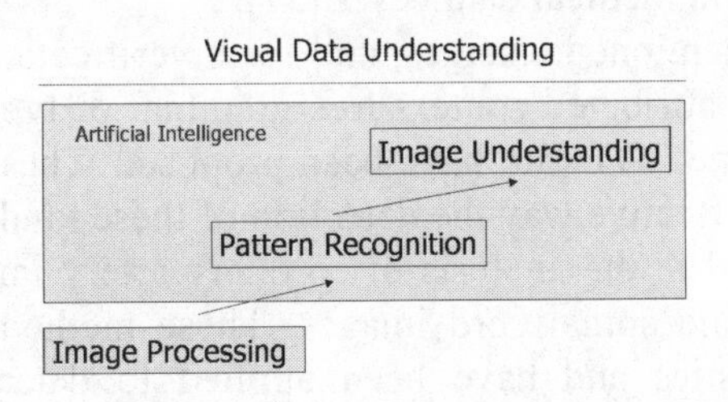

Fig. 4.1. Stages of image analysis in Visual Data Understanding systems

The chapter will discus in particular disease symptom recognition tasks for three selected types of medical images:

1. Analysis of coronary arteries seen on coronographic images [10, 17]. This analysis is aimed to discover the symptoms of the ischaemic heart disease.
2. Renal pelvis with ureters visible on urograms of these structures [18]. An analysis of urograms allows one to diagnose some lesions characteristic for hydronephrosis or extrarenal uraemia.
3. Pancreatic ducts visible on images obtained in the course of ERCP (Endoscopic Retrograde Cholangio-Pancreatography) examinations [1, 30]. In this case the objective of the analysis is early computer-aided diagnosis of neoplastic lesions and pancreatitis.
4. Spine and spinal cord visualised on NMR images. The objective is to detect and diagnose lesions that might evidence a whole range of various disease units (from numerous forms of inflammatory conditions to most serious cases of tumours)

The process of recognition will be based mainly on the use of context-free attributed grammars, languages of shape feature description as well as graph grammars used to recognise disease symptoms, which can occur in these organs. This type of recognition may not only support the diagnosis of disease lesions but it also constitutes intelligent information systems imitating the method of image interpretation and understanding as performed by qualified professionals.

Algorithms proposed in this chapter constitute a new proposal for an efficient and effective analysis of selected organ morphology, aimed to diagnose pathological lesions in them. They also expand current analysis techniques to a considerable degree by offering possibilities to specify the semantic content of images, which can support the diagnosis and further treatment directions. Moreover, they may also serve for a quick indexation and categorisation of disease units in medical data bases [37].

For a proper diagnosis of the mentioned changes, and for a verification of how advanced their level is, an attributed context-free grammar of type LR (1) and a graph grammar of type EDT [56] have been proposed. These grammars permit in an unusually effective way the detection of these kinds of irregularities and are also useful in the analysis of coronary artery images, urograms, pancreatograms and spinal cord images. These methods derive from mathematical linguistics and have been applied to detect changes in the width of different structures, visible in graphs. These graphs are obtained owing to the application of a straightening transformation at the stage of image pre-processing, which enables the production of straightened structure graphs, while preserving morphological lesions occurring in them.

The general methodology of application of syntactic pattern recognition for the creation of perceptual description for analysed structures and pathological signs is the following: first simple shape elements are defined, the general grammar description of the analysed organ is built. The bases for this description are a special kind of graph, tree or context-free grammars [40, 56]. Using the actual shape of organ in question we can obtain a description in the form of sequences of terminal symbols. Such sequences belong to the languages generated by the introduced grammar. The obtained description sentences are different for each lesion and for a healthy organ because every organ is unique. The main analysis and recognition of pathological signs are based on parsing algorithms, which analyse input sentences and reduce them to one of known categories. For each case of disease it is possible to obtain a unique parsing result, belonging to one of some classes. In the rare cases, from the diagnostic point of view, of equivalence of some classes it is also necessary to establish the final result of recognition by applying simple methods based on specially defined semantic procedures [34].

Furthermore, this type of recognition in its essence is an attempt to automate a specifically human understanding process of medical meaning of the implication of organ shapes on a digital image. It is based on a perception, in other words on a deeper understanding of the examined image.

The main advantage resulting from the use of the presented grammars is that they offer a possibility to detect, on the obtained width profiles, both concentric stenoses, revealed on a regular cross-section by the monotonous stenosis of the whole lumen, as well as eccentric stenoses revealed only on one side of the vessel. This property is especially useful for coronary artery diagnosis because it allows us to see whether the detected symptom is characteristic of stable angina pectoris in the case of concentric stenosis diagnosis, or unstable angina pectoris when an eccentric stenosis is revealed.

Further chapters will present algorithms of initial analysis of the discussed images as well as recognition methods together with examples of results of disease lesions recognition in coronary arteries, upper urinary tracts, pancreatic ducts and spinal cord.

4.2. Pre-processing Methods Designed to Process Selected Medical Images

4.2.1. A Need to Apply Medical Data Pre-processing

The recognition of the looked-for disease lesions on the discussed medical images conducted with the use of the syntactic methods of pattern recognition proposed in this book is possible only owing to prior preparation of the examined image in a very special and highly aimed way. This means that the application of syntactic methods of image analysis must be preceded by an application of a special operation sequence belonging to pre-processing of the examined images. Due to that the final objective of the analysis presented in this chapter will be to understand the essence of selected health problems connected with imminent myocardial infraction, urinary system artresia and pancreas failure. Thus the starting point for the analysis will be to visualise the pathological lesions of the respective organ shapes. Due to the need to eliminate various factors (e.g. individual variation) which change the **appearance** of the organs in question on an image and thus change the meaning of the contents of its imaging (e.g. pointing to the occurrence of symptoms of a given disease), we looked for such a form of pre-processing, which would retain information necessary to understand an image and at the same time eliminate information noise.

In tasks presented in this chapter we have the following examples of disturbing factors: the general course, size and shape as well as location of the analysed anatomical structures on the image. All those factors ensuing both from the anatomical features of body build of an individual as well as from the method used to take the particular X-ray photograph, influence strongly the shape of structures visible on the image. Yet they do not determine the evaluation of the image as such (that is the decision whether a given organ is healthy or if there are signs of pathology). A medical doctor aiming to understand the essence of a patient's ailment takes out those unimportant features and focuses his/her attention on details important for the diagnosis. In the examples discussed here those details are stenoses or dilations (sometimes also ramifications) of the appropriate vessels. This is why in the examples analysed here, pre-processing of the examined images has been directed at obtaining straightened (which means that the vessel course is independent of individual variations) and appropriately smoothed width diagrams of the vessel. They are the carrier of information necessary to **understand** if we are dealing with a healthy organ or one with pathological lesions. Later we shall see examples of such width diagrams obtained as a result of pre-processing of the analysed coronary arteries, ureters, main pancreatic ducts, and spinal cord. Those diagrams are subsequently approximated by means of segments of an open polygon, and segments are characterised by means of symbols of a selected grammar. Owing to this we obtain a description of the examined organ shape, limiting considerably the representation of those fragments (which usually take a lot of space on the image), which can be considered to be physiologically correct. It visualises all pathological lesions of interest to us, occurring on the examined structures.

The above-presented concept of pre-processing medical images prepared for the analysis process, aimed to finish by an automatic understanding of the essence of pathological lesions shown on them, contains many important and difficult details; their solution was necessary for the functioning of the method described here. We shall comment shortly on some of those numerous problems associated with image pre-processing that have been undertaken and solved before it was possible to describe attempts at automatic understanding of the medical content and the essence of information about deformations visible on images.

First let us emphasise that in order to achieve the aimed-for objectives it was necessary to obtain width diagrams of the analysed structures in such a way that they visualise both the concentric and eccentric stenoses. It is possible to achieve this objective owing to the application, at the pre-processing stage, of an approach to determining the central line and creating a width diagram slightly different than the ones proposed by other researchers [9, 17]. The conducted research has shown that in order to obtain the central line (axis) of the analysed vessel, rather than the operation of morphological erosion of the binarised vessel proposed by some researchers, or (performed by a specialist) manual positioning of the location of the said line, we should use a different technique which gives much better results. Similar research has demonstrated that in the course of attempts at automatic understanding of pathological lesions of the examined organ structure and of deformations of the analysed organ shape indicating those, the best results are obtained when the reference line is a curvilinear axis of the vessel. This axis can be laid out by the method of skeletonisation of the analysed anatomical structures used by the authors. The method is based on an appropriately modified Pavlidis algorithm [49]. The said method is efficient in calculations and the central line obtained in its result, with precisely central location in relation to its walls (also in the case in which they are pathologically deformed), creates a certain path along with width profiles determined [24].

If we take a numerically **straightened** axis line of the analysed vessel for our reference point then we obtain diagrams of its unilaterals (the so-called top and bottom or left and right). Those diagrams are obtained owing to the use of a specialist algorithm of the so-called straightening transformation prepared by the authors; it allows us to obtain width diagrams of the analysed structures together with morphological lesions occurring in them [27]. Those diagrams are subsequently approximated with a polygon, which constitutes the basis for the further-discussed automatic understanding process of pathological deformations of the analysed organs visualised on images.

4.2.2. Recommended Stages of Medical Data Pre-processing

To summarise the above-said we can say that the following – below specified operations – should be conducted in the course of pre-processing of the examined images (in square brackets are references to bibliography items supplying all necessary technical details relating both to the algorithms and details of implementation):

1. Segmentation and filtering of the analysed images (in the examples of coronarographic, ERCP and urogram images analysed here) [3, 9, 17, 21].
2. Skeletonisation of the analysed structures of selected vessels visualised on images, e.g. on images of coronary arteries, main pancreatic ducts, ureters, and spinal cords [25, 41].
3. Analysis of real and verification of apparent[1] skeleton ramifications [26].
4. Smoothing the skeleton by averaging its elements [24].
5. The application of a specially prepared straightening transformation, transforming the external contour of the examined structures in a two-dimensional space to the form of 2D width diagrams, visualising contours of the ‘numerically straightened' organ. This transformation retains all morphological details of the analysed structures (in particular their deformations and pathological lesions). For this reason it is a convenient

[1] Due to the fact that ramifications in the skeleton appearing as a result of skeletonisation can occur as artefacts in the course of thinning out irregularities occurring at the external edges of the examined structures or they can be real ramifications, as it is the case in for example in pancreatic ducts, it is necessary to conduct an analysis of those ramifications allowing to remove the apparent ramifications and to determine the order of real ramifications.

starting point for further analysis of shape feature properties of the analysed structure and for detecting such deformations (with the use of syntactic methods of pattern recognition). This constitutes the basis for an automatic understanding of pathological lesions' nature and for a diagnosis of the disease under consideration [32].

Recognition and automatic understanding of the looked-for lesions of organ shapes with the use of syntactic methods of pattern recognition is possible owing to a prior application of the specified sequence of operations, which together constitute the previously mentioned image pre-processing stage. Details relating to individual stages of pre-processing the analysed images were discussed at length in (above-quoted) publications of the authors. They will also be demonstrated on examples and in further chapters of this book. Those stages have been specified also on Figure 4.2.

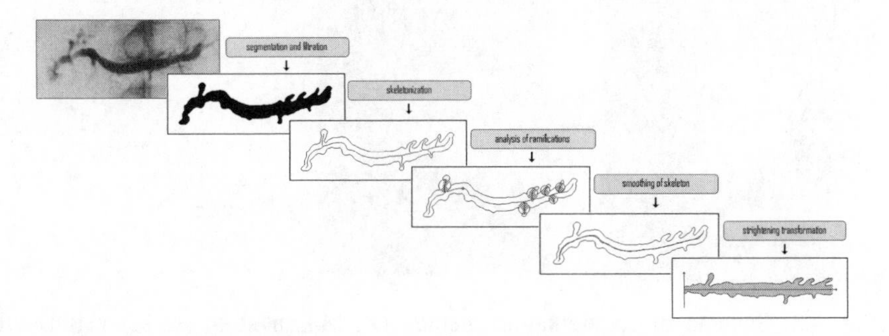

Fig. 4.2. Operations conducted in the course of pre-processing of the examined images. At the top is the original image of pancreatic duct showing symptoms of chronic inflammation. At the bottom a diagram of the pancreatic duct contours with visible morphological lesions

4.2.3. Segmentation and Filtering of Images

One of the first steps of initial analysis of the discussed medical images is their segmentation. It allows us to extract from a complete image of the examined organs the contour of elements important from the diagnosis point of view (in the examples shown here those are vessels filled with contrast fluid). Simultaneously, excessive morphological elements of the examined organ and of other anatomical and non-anatomical structures visualised on, which together belong to the background of the image under consideration, are suppressed (often they are more contrasting than the examined vessel, in particular when the elements are bones of the vertebral column or fragments of a probe with contrast).

A specialist threshold algorithm proposed in papers [21, 40] has been used for the segmentation of all X-ray images analysed in this chapter. This algorithm has proved [21] its considerable usefulness as the optimal method for ERCP image binarisation. It has been assumed therefore that this algorithm will be just as effective for the segmentation of coronographic images and urograms. Experimental research has confirmed this assumption.

This algorithm has been described in a formal and complete way in papers quoted in [21]; in this chapter we shall only characterise qualitatively its concept by stating that it operates in the following way (see Figure 4.3.).

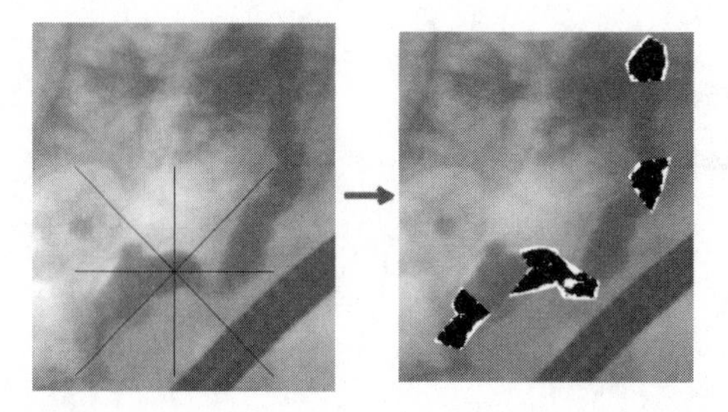

Fig. 4.3. Scheme of segmentation method (Z. Mikrut et al. A METHOD OF LINEAR 'STAR-SECTIONS' APPLIED FOR OBJECT SEPARATION IN ERCP IMAGES (ICIP'96, Lausanne))

In the course of binarisation of the analysed image, the looked-for edge points of the examined structure (isolated vessel) are determined based on an analysis of derivatives of eight scalar functions. Those functions have been defined as densitometric profiles for eight directional straight lines. Directional straight lines form a symmetrical star of canonical directions and they originate in the so-called central analysis points (selected automatically in subsequent analysis steps). All points belonging to their direct or indirect environment are taken into consideration in selecting the successive central points of analysis. The first central point of the analysis must be indicated manually (so that the algorithm knows which anatomic structure it should separate from among many visible ones). If the process of filling of the analysed vessel with the contrasting fluid has not been performed correctly – or in cases in which the advanced disease process has led to a very considerable stricture of the vessel lumen in some of its segments, then, on the roentgenogram, the outline of the examined vessel can be discontinued. In this case there is a need to show manually to the binarising software at least one initial central point of analysis in every well visible segment of the examined anatomic structure.

Densitometric functions introduced here specify changes of the grey-scale levels of successive points of the image located on the defined directional straight lines, depending on their distance from the central analysis point, currently under consideration. The point, in which there is a big negative value of the derivative of the analysed densitometric function, is presumed to be an edge point. This decision is additionally verified in context (based on neighbouring points among which there should also be previously discovered edge points). In this way image segmentation and separation (as well as binarisation) of the examined vessel's interior image takes place in a dispersed way (in many segments of the depicted vessel simultaneously): first in those areas, in which natural contrasting of the vessel is particularly good compared to the tissue surrounding it, and only later in areas in which the contrast is inferior and where it is possible to use context information resulting from the known, previously extracted contour fragments. Details relating to the binarisation procedure shortly described here (a procedure which turned out to be very efficient) are too complicated to quote them here in their entirety. They can be found in the following works: [21].

It is worth adding that this complex binarisation procedure has to be applied only in the case of particularly difficult images (for example a pancreatic duct inaccurately filled with contrast with an overlaying vertebral column image). In the case of other, simpler medical images, it is possible to approach the segmentation task and to discover the edges of the analysed vessels by means of the subtractive method of combining original images with images that underwent high-pass filtering. Next the method of gradient analysis is applied to the result of this operation; its aim is to identify the edges.

Just as effective, especially for determining the edges of coronary arteries, is the method of high-pass temporal filtering [17]. The filtering is conducted in a situation in which in order to separate the looked-for structure we use a whole sequence of images registered during one coronary arteries contrasting procedure. This type of filtering allows one to isolate the looked-for structure based on a change of contrasts occurring at the passage from one image of a given sequence to another. We use the fact that anatomical structures, which are not subject to any movement or contrasting while a sequence of such images is taken (theoretically) generate information with temporal frequency equal to 0 Hz. Although some small movement of those objects, caused by the patient's breathing while images are taken, can also generate information changing in time (diagnostically unimportant) for those anatomical structures, their frequency will be lower than the typical frequency range connected with heart rate, amounting to 1–2 Hz. It is sufficient therefore to discriminate by removing sequences of immovable images (or moving slowly) in order to obtain the effect of extracting the (further analysed) anatomical structures of interest to us. The above-mentioned frequency filters are used for this very purpose. They liquidate all elements of the image represented in the frequency domain by frequency component below 1 Hz. The general concept of filtering is the following:

Let I_j stand for a sequence composed of j images. It is possible to determine for any j moment an integrated filtering mask M_j, based on summing up some of the so far obtained images, e.g.:

$$M_j = I_{j-1} + I_{j-2} + \dots + I_{j-n}$$

Where $n \times \delta t$ is a temporal interval for obtaining n images, δt is the time of obtaining two successive images (1/30s is the standard). The image components represented by temporal frequencies below $1/n \times \delta t$ can be removed by simple deduction of M_j from the last image of the I_j sequence.

The above-described binarisation methods are usually sufficient; however, they are not fit for the segmentation of CT (computer tomography) images, most often binarised by means of methods based on the examination of volume increase of the analysed organs [55].

Images of the examined medical structures, binarised in this or another way are then subject to the procedure of edge smoothing. It is necessary because due to the (usually) not very good contrast of the medical images under consideration, the binarisation procedures of those images often produce irregular edges of the isolated objects, which should then be smoothed by performing the averaging or median filtering. Usually the application of those simple operations on the binarised image suffices entirely to remove all irregularities occurring on the external edges of the examined objects [28]. By means of notation commonly adopted in image algebra both filtering operations can be described with the following formulae:

The averaging filtering operation: $b(y) = \frac{1}{n} \sum_{x \in N(y)} a(x)$, for $\forall y \in a$

Where $\boldsymbol{a}$ stands for the prime input image, $\boldsymbol{b}$ stands for the output image obtained as a result of the operation of averaging the neighbourhood of successive points, $\boldsymbol{a(x)}$ stands for the grey level of point with the $\boldsymbol{x}$ coordinate (where $x \in Z^2$) of the input image, ***b(y)*** stands for the grey level of the point with the ***y*** coordinate of the output image, ***n*** stands for the number of points belonging to the *N(y)* neighbourhood of a given point *y* ($n=card(N(y)\ \forall y \in Z^2$).

Similarly, the median filtering operation can be recorded as:
$b(y) = med\{a(x), x \in N(y)\}$, for $\forall y \in a$

In the above-given notation, the *med* function is a function specifying the median value for the selected neighbourhood of the a(x) point (usually this is a neighbourhood whose size is 3 x 3 pixel covering 9 or 5 points).

4.2.4. Skeletonisation of the Analysed Anatomical Structures

The next stage of the binarised roentgenogram analysis is the **skeletonisation** of anatomical structures visualised in the course of the segmentation. It can be conducted in many different ways due to the fact that literature describes a big number of algorithms, which can be used for this purpose. In every case, as a result of the skeletonisation we obtain a central line of the thinned out object; additionally the line should be parallel to the external borders and its thickness should be even. All known skeletonisation algorithms meet the above-listed postulates but the quality of skeletons obtained varies (see the Figure 4.4) and some skeletons are not fit at all for the purposes, which are intended for them in the framework of the described concept of automatic medical image understanding.

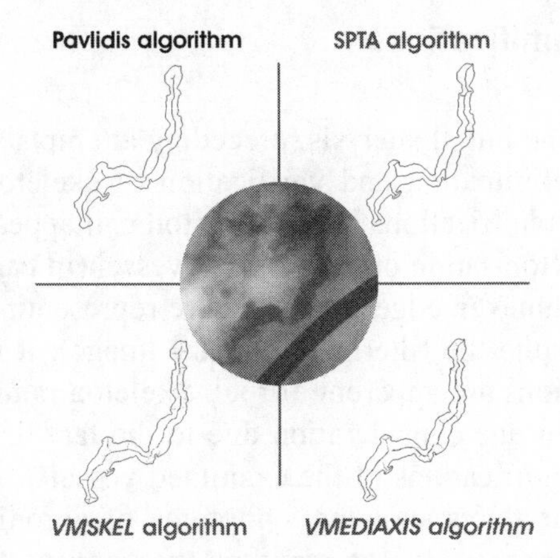

Fig. 4.4. Results of skeletonisation the ducts with pancreas cancer using various algorithms

By means of comparative research we have also found [26] that for the purpose of skeletonisaton of structures interesting for us it is possible to use the Pavlidis skeletonisation algorithm, as one of the best from among a number of methods analysed for this purpose [27]. The main advantage of this algorithm is the generation of continuous, very regular and smooth skeletons, characterised by unitary width and genuinely central location in relation to the contours of the thinned out structure. Moreover, the Pavlidis skeleton lines are only slightly shortened at the ends during the analysis; this constitutes an additional benefit of this method as compared to other often-used algorithms. An extremely important advantage of this method selected, important from the point of view of effectiveness of further skeleton structure analysis, is the fact that in this method we get the smallest number of apparent side ramifications in the skeleton. Apparent side ramifications of the skeleton, which appear as a result of skeletonisation of those vessel images on which there are some small irregularities of the contour, constitute a considerable obstacle during attempts at automatic understanding of the examined vessel shape. They also complicate significantly the task of understanding the meaning of this very shape (rather than a different one) – as seen from the viewpoint of the assessment of the examined organ form and a diagnosis proposal.

Figures 4.2 and 4.4 show examples of the result of a skeletonisation operation on binary pancreatic duct images.

4.2.5. Analysis of Skeleton Ramifications

The next important step of the image initial analysis, preceding attempts at its automatic recognition, is the elimination and verification of skeleton ramifications. Due to the fact that ramifications in the skeleton can appear as artefacts resulting from the skeletonisation of the selected vessel (in particular in the case of irregular and uneven edges of the figure representing the examined organ, occurring despite the filtering of binary image), it is necessary to check if the ramifications are apparent or real. Skeleton ramifications cannot be rejected without due consideration due to the fact that they can be the skeletons of real ramifications of the examined vessel – as it often is the case with pancreatic ducts showing symptoms of chronic pancreatitis. What is more, if there are ramifications, then they constitute an important premise in the process of automatic reasoning aimed at understanding image features. In this situation the simple method of cutting off ramifications can be used to eliminate apparent ramifications only in the case in which they occur as a result of skeletonisation of irregular ureter, coronary artery or spinal cord contours (that is, of course, with the assumption that we limit our interest only to the anatomical structures listed in the beginning of this chapter). In other cases (again, with the assumption of a limited scope of analysed cases, relating only to **some** ureter images) at the pre-processing stage it is necessary to conduct a more detailed analysis of such ramifications in order to determine if they are important from the viewpoint of further diagnosis or if they constitute typical artefacts. In the case of ERCP images it is possible that there will be skeletons of real side ramifications of a given vessel, whose analysis (relating to the location, number, shapes and sizes as well as the so-called order) is necessary, for example, to determine the degree to which chronic inflammation is advanced. This is why while preparing the pre-processing methods for the examined medical images; we prepared a special procedure for analysing side ramifications in those images. It allows to detect and locate in individual sections of the pancreatic duct, every ramification discovered as well as to determine its order and to verify whether that is an apparent ramification, appearing as the artefact of skeletonisation. An example of image of pancreatic duct with ramifications and a schematic idea governing the operation of the verification method has been presented on Figure 4.5.

The original methods of elimination of side ramifications in the skeletons of pancreatic ducts prepared by the authors have been described in the work [29]. The operation of this method has been described in detail in the paper [37]. Its iteration implementation allows us to determine precisely the number of real ramifications of the 1st and 2nd order occurring on the image; the said analysis can be conducted separately in individual segments of the pancreatic duct. Information obtained on this pre-processing stage can be used for the determination of the degree to which chronic pancreatitis or pancreas neoplasm are advanced; it can be used also to localise the inflammation process.

Developing this idea we should say that in order to conduct a complete analysis of the type of side ramifications occurring, we should apply a sequence of two algorithms pre-processing the analysed images. First we use the skeleton ramification algorithm, which allows for a precise determination if the examined ramification is real or apparent. The algorithm verifying (and rejecting) apparent ramifications in the skeleton is based on an examination of the degree of belonging of the neighbourhood of a selected (usually central) point of the 'suspect' ramification in the outline of the examined structure (e.g. inside the pancreatic duct lumen). If the skeleton ramification visibly goes beyond the outline of the duct itself, it is treated as a real ramification. In the other case we can suspect that the side ramification of the skeleton has been generated by the skeletonisation algorithm, 'provoked' by a specific course of edge line of the examined vessel. Further steps of the described method of apparent side ramification verification have been presented in Table 4.1.

Having verified that we are dealing with real ramifications we shall relate to the next algorithm owing to which those ramifications (that is only the ones, which have been verified as real ramifications) are located in individual parts of the pancreatic duct, e.g. in the head, body and tail: based on the specified for this purpose percentage length proportions of every of those parts, as compared to the length of the entire pancreatic duct. The said proportions have been specified based on topographic relations of the pancreas to the vertebral column; the method according to which they have been determined has been presented in [29]. It is worth adding that in the task of automatic understanding of ERCP images discussed here, the determination of such correct proportions of individual pancreatic duct segments was necessary to make the correct diagnosis. This resulted from the fact that the diagnosis of this group of medical problems depends strongly on the place in which morphological lesions occur – they play the role of disease symptoms along the axis of the examined vessel, in this case the main pancreatic duct.

Table 4.1 Stages of the algorithm of apparent skeleton ramifications verification with the use of the circular neighbourhood method

Stage	Operation performed
1	Determination of the length of the analysed ramification
2	Circumscribing a circle in the central point of the ramification with radius equal to its distance from the prime point of the ramification
3	Determination of the quantity of two ratios defined in the following way: Number_ points_background:=number of points from the background of the image belonging to the circumscribed circle number_all_points:= number of all points belonging to the circumscribed circle
4	Verification of the condition: if (Number_ points_background < 0.1* number_all_points OR Number_ points_background < 20) then (the examined ramification is apparent); else (examined ramification is real);

the number 20 in the if instruction condition stands for the minimal threshold established by means of experiments.

The operation of this method is based on the fact that the external edges of morphological convexities and cysts are more circular and filled than the sharp and narrow edges of real ramifications. Thus greater erosion of apparent ramification in the course of skeletonisation leads to a situation, in which such ramifications go deeper into the skeletonised duct, as shown on Figure 4.5. This leads to a situation in which circles circumscribed in this way are contained completely or almost completely in the examined organs (e.g. pancreatic ducts); this constitutes the basis for a quick and relatively unmistakeable reasoning. The said relates to various vessels, not only the pancreatic ducts analysed here. Thus, the above-given simple, intuitive and computationally effective ratio can find numerous applications in the assessment of ramification existence in various anatomical structures (or lack thereof). An implementation example of the verification algorithm of apparent skeleton ramification with the circular neighbourhood has been presented on Figure 4.5.

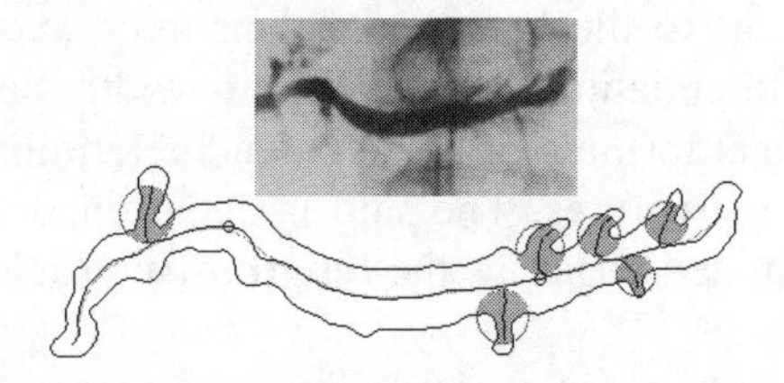

Fig. 4.5. Example of skeleton analysis ramifications in the main pancreatic duct. The figure shows circular neighbourhood of the central points of skeleton ramifications. Borders of individual parts of the pancreatic duct are shown with small circles on the main skeleton line; from the left: head, body and tail. On the main skeleton line shown in grey, we indicated also the line obtained as a result of skeleton smoothing with the averaging method

The iteration implementation of the algorithm presented here allows one to determine precisely the number and place of occurrence on the image of real ramifications of the 1st and 2nd order. This has an application mainly in individual parts of the pancreatic duct due to the fact that in this very case this piece of information can be further used to determine the degree to which chronic pancreatitis or pancreas neoplasm is advanced. However, in the case of coronary arteries, spinal cord, and the analysed sections of ureters – these are only the examples of the anatomical structures analysed here – the above-described algorithm allows one to remove excessive apparent ramifications if the skeletonisation algorithm produces such 'artefacts' due to the complicated shape of the organ with disease lesions.

4.2.6. Smoothing skeletons of the analysed anatomical structures

As a result of the recognition of real and the elimination of apparent side ramifications in the analysed vessel skeleton, only the main skeleton lines are transferred to further analysis. They can be very strongly deformed and interfered so before beginning the analysis and attempting to understand the feature shapes of the examined objects, they are smoothed. The skeletons are smoothed by means of averaging their successive elements in relation to points belonging to their environment. This process of current filtering is executed for every skeleton point analysed at the moment. The size of the neighbourhood defined for all skeleton points should be the same and – as test research has demonstrated – it should be equal to half of the average width of the examined object [29]. Since, in the case of some anatomical structures, doubts can arise as to the location of their main axes, thus causing difficulties with differentiating between their width and length, it is useful to apply a numerical formula of the averaged determination of the 'average width' of those structures. The said is determined as the quotient of the **field** of the examined organ to the **length** of its skeleton.

An exemplary result of smoothing the main skeleton line of the pancreatic duct with the averaging method has been shown on Figure 4.5.

Along the thus smoothed skeletons we shall execute the **straightening transformation**, very important for all issues considered here. The origin of its name is that it evens (straightens) the course of the main axis of the examined organ; assuming that usually its curvatures and the general location depend on idiosyncratic features of the 'organ owner' as well as the technical method in which the image of the analysed organ was taken (e.g. the angle of the X-ray tube and the radiation detector used while the image is taken with the use of X-rays). The straightening transformation, by eliminating factors of individual variation in their majority not useful for further reasoning, retains relatively faithfully the external contours of the examined organs. On this basis it is possible (in the examples analysed here) to take diagnostic decisions. The general, the objective of this transformation is to eliminate excessive variation features of the medical images analysed here (and subject to attempts of automatic understanding). In this chapter, due to the fact that examples analysed here relate mainly to such problems, in which the medical problem can be characterised by describing the deformation of the edge line of the organs under consideration, the general idea of the straightening transformation has been reduced to the process of obtaining width diagrams of the objects under consideration (coronary vessels, pancreatic ducts, spine or ureters). Simultaneously those diagrams retain and expose those morphological lesions, which can be included into symptoms which in an unambiguous way certify some disease processes in the examined organs. Width profile diagrams (symmetric or asymmetric), which are basically a 1D representation of the 3D phenomenon of pathological deformation of the examined organ shall be the starting point for the recognition and morphological analysis of those objects' shapes. The analysis will be performed with the use of syntactic methods of pattern recognition. The process of conversion of polimorphic deformation of object shape into an unambiguous diagnostic decision shall be identified with the key concept for this book, the concept of understanding the shapes of biological objects analysed here.

4.2.7. Transformation Straightening the External Contours of Analysed Objects

The topic of this chapter will be a presentation of details of the algorithm defined above as the straightening transformation. This algorithm, operating based on sequences of geometrical image transformation and transforming the external edge (contour) of the examined organ from the space of a complete (although already pre-processed) 2D image, has the objective to eliminate insignificant factors of image variability (originating mainly from the patient's individual features) and to transform a complex 2D organ shape (in itself difficult to describe and interpret) to the form of a 1D diagram. Diagrams obtained in this way (usually three: the upper profile, the lower profile and the symmetrical profile) will present the contours of the numerically 'straightened' organs. The essence of the usefulness of the above-mentioned profiles is that they abstract from factors strongly influencing the imaging shape but which from the diagnostic point of view are not very important. They 'concentrate' the attention of algorithms undertaking the attempt to understand images automatically on details of the external contour important from the diagnostic point of view: with all morphological formations which can occur on them, e.g. side ramifications or the bisection of the analysed structure, external contour convexity or visible stenoses or dilation of the lumen (*dimension*) of the analysed vessel.

The main advantage of the presented later method, i.e. representation of the analysed object shape using 1D results of its straightening transformation is that the straightening transformation retains all occurring morphological lesions. This means that on a 1D diagram – the outcome of the straightening transformation – we can find traces of all morphological details occurring in the analysed organ or in the analysed anatomical structure; those can be both lesions that lie within physiological norms and lesions which are clearly pathological ones. Despite the originally (on source images) morphologically very complex manifestation of different variants of the lesions under consideration, they are relatively simple on 1D diagrams resulting from the straightening transformation. This in turn enables their further analysis and diagnosis with the use of relatively simple methods, e.g. syntactic methods of pattern recognition proposed in this book.

It is worth adding that this transformation has passed its practical examination: it was used to diagnose diseases of organs such as pancreas based on analyses of X-ray images originating from ERCP examinations. It was also used to analyse the state of coronary vessels and (in the context of completely different diseases) for an assessment of the upper urinary tracts, as well as for the meaning analysis of spinal cord lesions. According to the authors of this book, the potential possibilities of the transformation described here are not exhausted yet. There is an additional possibility to use the proposed 'straightening transformation' algorithm for 3D analysis and for the modelling of spatially complex anatomical structures of such human body internal areas as abdominal cavity organs or the reconstruction of the bronchial tree; this can aid in diagnosing many other diseases, e.g. colon polyp or lung neoplasm.

The straightening transformation algorithm is *de facto* an algorithm of geometric transformation of the external contours of flat imaging of the analysed anatomical structures, in practice executed by subsequent rotation of all contour points of the organ around the successively determined points of a geometric axis (skeleton) of the organ. This algorithm is quite complex; it was described in detail in [29], therefore it is easy to reproduce on any computer and for any type of images. On 1D diagrams obtained as a result of the straightening transformation we can see shape features of the external borders of the vessel under consideration, the most important points with regards to further processing aimed at automatic understanding of image contents. This can be used, *inter alia,* (although not uniquely) for automatic disease diagnosing. The above-described methodology can also find its application in automatic indexation of multimedia data basis conducted in such a way, so that the registered records are grouped and addressed with regards to the concrete morphological lesions occurring in them. This will result in that searching for a given patient's record could be performed in reply to a query of the following type: 'show all cases with similar morphological lesions.'

In the method version described in this book, the classification, grouping and automatic recognition of medical images can be executed based on quite simple morphological criteria only: the type and character of disease lesions manifested on the external contours of the analysed anatomical structures. Exemplary results of obtaining the straightened width diagrams for the images analysed in this book, together with morphological lesions occurring in them, shall be presented in further chapters when concrete tasks of analysing various types of the images examined here will be described. It is worth adding, however, that the method presented here can be used (after appropriate generalisation) for attempts of automatic recognition of medical structures visualised with the state-of-the-art 3D techniques.

4.2.8. Straightening Transformation Algorithm

After a general description of the straightening transformation, now time has come to present it in more detail. Using the notation of the simplified C language, the **straightening transformation** algorithm can be, in a simplified version, recorded in the following way:

```
contour_straightening_algorithm()
        {
creating the representation of the object contour;

/* creation of transformed (e.g. 'straightened') object edges in relation to the skeleton */
for every skeleton point
  {
  determination of directional straight line crossing this point;
  determination of straight line for measuring the width of the examined object;
  determination of points where the contour crosses the width measuring
straight line;
  determination of location of those points in relation to the straight line;
  rotation of the determined contour points around the skeleton point under
consideration by angle opposite to the inclination angle of the measuring straight
line in relation to the OY axis;
  }
/*ordering, that is 'linearisation' of the obtained tables with contour coordinates */

sorting contour points;
removing excessive points of the straightened contour;
```

correcting the continuity of the obtained width diagram;
}

The operation of contour points determination on a given object does not cause considerable problems and it is executed in the course of one image viewing. We should make it clear that the term contour (edge) point will stand for every point with at least one neighbour from the object background. With all edge points of the considered organ at our disposal and the central line of the binary graphic object representing it (obtained as a result of skeletonisation) we can, point by point, rotate (numerically) edge points which are on the intersection of the figure with the measuring straight line, defined as the straight line perpendicular to the so-called directional straight line. The measuring straight line is used to measure the object width, determined in the skeleton point currently under consideration. The directional straight line is necessary to show the direction of the skeleton line course of the examined figure in the currently analysed point of that skeleton. Determination of the exact direction of this line requires a determination of the direction of the skeleton course; this can be obtained by means of the tangent method or the secant method. In the algorithms described here we use the secant method, as illustrated below. These operations (that is the determination of the direction of the directional straight line, followed by constructing a measuring line on its basis and determination of points where it intersects with the contour of the analysed figure) are executed successively for every skeleton point. The results of measuring the distance between contour points and the figure axis along the selected sequence of measuring straight lines are stacked on a 1D diagram whose vertical axis is described by the number of the successive points tracked along the figure axis. A consequent implementation of the steps described here leads in consequence to the appearance of a new 1D width diagram of the analysed vessel, similar to its straightened contour – hence the name 'straightening transformation.'

We should note, of course, that the above-given shortened description simplifies a number of issues. In many cases in real application the analysed anatomical structures (and in particular their skeletons) are very often characterised by numerous multi-directional curvatures, which result in that during the determination of successive measuring straight lines, the points in which they intersect with the internal contour are the same; therefore in the establishment of the straightened contour the co-ordinates of those points must by considered a number of times. This does not change the general idea of the fully implemented method described above.

The reason why we explained what kind of detailed problems have to be solved in the method implementation will be presented below: the rule governing the determination of the measuring straight line and the directional straight line. The task of determination of directional straight lines crossing the successive skeleton points is in fact based on a sequence of lines tangent to the organ axis – in a situation in which the axis changes its direction a number of times. The method applied is based on a prior determination of secant of the organ axis and a construction of a straight line horizontal to the secant, located precisely in the considered skeleton point. The secant representing the skeleton direction in a given point is based on two neighbouring skeleton points (in relation to the currently examined point), symmetrically distant by a certain determined distance from the point, in which the directional straight line should be placed. The support points of the secant determine the neighbourhood of the application point of the directional straight line (points marked as B on Figure 4.6); the neighbourhood determines the location of the determined directional straight line (straight line C on Figure 4.6).

The conducted research has demonstrated that the optimum size of the determined neighbourhood should be approximately equal to the object width (that is the vessel under consideration) determined in the previous step of the algorithm (in the previous skeleton point) [29]. This strategy allows to obtain a very equal and regular distribution of the measuring straight lines determined and used to determine the vessel width in its individual points. After establishing the inclination direction of the directional straight line crossing a given environment, we should translate the straight line in such a way that it crosses precisely the currently analysed skeleton point. At that point it is a good approximation (not very sensitive to local axis surging) of the tangent to the organ skeleton (straight line D on Figure 4.6).

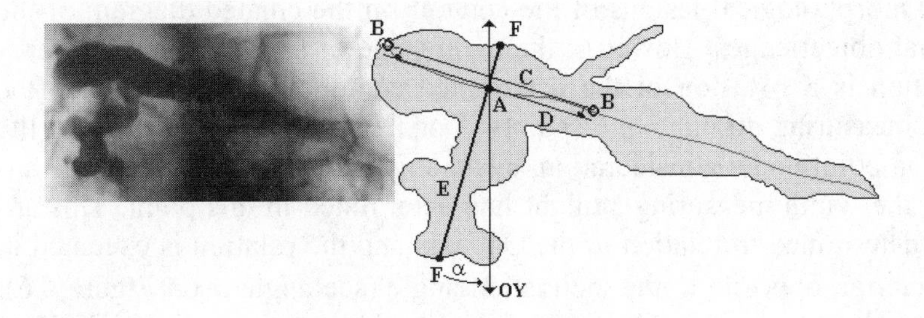

Fig. 4.6. The method of geometric transformation leading to the determination of the examined structure's width diagram. Point A stands for the currently analysed skeleton point in which the object width is established. Point B determines the neighbourhood of point A, which allows to establish the directional straight line C. Straight line D has come into existence as a result of directional straight line C translation in such a way that it crosses the current skeleton point A. On the other hand, the straight line E, is a width measuring straight line, perpendicular to the straight line D. Points F are points at which the width measuring straight line intersects with the object's external contour. Those points are rotated around point A by angle α (established by straight line E and the OY axis), which leads to 'straightening' of the object

The next step is the determination of the width measuring straight line in the skeleton point currently under consideration, as a straight line perpendicular to the previously established directional straight line crossing this point (straight line E on Figure 4.6). After the determination of such a straight line it is necessary to find points at which it intersects the object contour; this is performed by viewing all edge points and verification whether any of them meet the equation of the width straight line. It is worth noticing that in the case of occurrence of real side ramifications of the analysed vessel it is possible that **many** points of object edge intersection will be found (analysed image of the separated fragment of the examined organ) as a result of which the diagram of its 'straightened' contour in a general case is not a function!

After all the intersection points of measuring the straight line with the object contour are determined, their location in relation to the skeleton is defined, in particular with regards to the previously established directional straight line at a given skeleton point. A correct location of points is extremely important from the point of view of the representation correctness for all morphological lesions of the contour on the created diagram of the external object edges. However, the main stage of the straightening transformation is a **rotation** of the determined contour points located on the width measuring straight line (points F on Figure 4.6) in relation to the skeleton point under consideration, by an angle equal to the inclination angle of the width measuring straight line determined in this point. This angle is determined in relation to the OY axis and the rotation is executed in the direction opposite to the inclination angle (see angle α on Figure 4.6). As a result of execution of this rotation all width measuring straight lines are vertical on the constructed diagram; this in turn results in that the previously obtained contour points marked on them create together a straightened diagram of external edges of the analysed object.

For the determined points of straightened contours it is necessary to conduct the following operations:

1. Line sorting so that it is possible to go successively through all points of the determined edge, together with the contour of the morphological lesions visualised on the image. This operation is indispensable due to a need to establish a straight line and to represent in an ambiguous way the newly established contour for the needs of our further analysis.
2. Decreasing the thickness of the obtained contour to one pixel with the use of standard skeletonisation algorithms. This operation is necessary due to the fact that after the process of extraction of edge points on individual measuring straight lines there are clusters of a few pixels in some contour points.
3. Enhancing the continuity of the obtained diagram using the approximation of successive point sequences by straight line segments with appropriately selected inclination and location.

Analysis of this diagram, rather than the original organ image, has a number of advantages. The diagram eliminates variation factors connected both with features of individual build of given patient's examined organ (it limits the influence of individual variation onto the process of further **meaning** analysis of specified shape features found on the examined object). The diagram is also (owing to the sequential ordering of its points) a 1D structure, representing all basic features of the considered 2D image, which facilitates significantly its linguistic description and further analysis based on syntactic methods. Most importantly, on diagrams constructed according to the methods described here, it is possible to identify and describe precisely all morphological lesions, which in reality occur on the external contours of the diagnosed anatomical structures. Due to the fact that those details of the shape of the analysed images are (in the here-analysed exemplary problems) most important from the point of view of the image understanding process and for its whole further diagnosis, therefore the process of automatic reasoning based only on width diagrams of the selected vessel separated from the organ image can be fully equivalent to the process of reasoning conducted on the basis of the complete organ image – it is considerably simple and cheaper from the point of view of computer implementation.

The enumerated operations result in that the obtained contour diagrams have a line representation and unitary width; moreover they are deprived of discontinuity points. An exemplary result of obtaining a straightened width diagram of the pancreatic duct together with the occurring morphological lesions has been presented on Figure 4.2.

4.2.9. Basic Advantages of the Proposed Pre-processing Method

The conducted research has confirmed great usefulness of the described method of geometric contour transformation in computer analysis and support to automatic medical diagnosis, conducted based on an analysis of various types of medical images, including ERCP roentgenograms, coronarograms and urograms [29].

The algorithm described here is appropriate both to obtain unilateral width diagrams (separately upper and separately lower) as well as bilateral (summary) width diagrams of the examined structures; they guarantee that in both cases simultaneously all pathological disease lesions existing on the external edges of the examined vessel will be exposed. Mirroring such lesions, occurring as a result of using the contour diagram method proposed here, enables their precise recognition e.g. with the use of syntactic pattern recognition methods.

The main advantage of the above-described method of pre-processing the analysed images is that in the case of syntactic method application for further analysis of those images for image understanding and recognition, there is no need to define for them 2D graphic primitives with a complicated form – which is one of barriers to the development of linguistic methods in image-related tasks. We shall explain that in more detail. If there were no pre-processing described above, the implementation of the postulate of syntactic image analysis would force us to detect and determine a whole set of the so-called primitive components in an image (called also graph primitives) which play the role of lexical components in the created and used graph grammars ('letters' or tokens). Those components serve first of all to describe features of shapes of the recognised objects. In the example analysed here they describe such features and geometric symptoms, which allow the differentiation of every image of a healthy organ (which looks slightly different in every human being) from any images of organs with signs of pathological lesions (which also can take various forms, even if the disease that deforms the organ is the same). The alphabet of such graphic patterns and image elements in primitive (non-processed) images would have to take into consideration any and all individual variations, complex spatial location of the analysed structures, various possible forms of pathology, etc. Every of those features can take hundreds of possible forms and their mutual location is totally unforeseeable. The said location can be additionally changed, for example as a result of change of the patients' body location while the photo is taken, also in consequence of variable penetration of the contrast into the examined vessels as well as variable features of the equipment used to obtain the image.

A set of those difficulties, of which some have just been enumerated, is the reason why we can frequently encounter an opinion that it is impossible to apply effectively syntactic method to recognise the looked-for disease lesions on typical medical images. It turns out that the majority of the above-listed problems can be avoided if the image syntactic analysis process is preceded by the above-described image pre-processing (or another one adequate to the situation). Graph primitives, diagnostically useful and extremely difficult to define for the original images, turn out to be easy to define and use if the syntactic analysis is conducted on diagrams obtained as a result of pre-processing. This thesis will be substantiated (below) by a demonstration of how simple a set of lexical elements can be used for the creation of a syntactic description for a wide class of medical images – after they are pre-processed in accordance with the above presented pre-processing rules.

4.3. Making Lexical Elements for the Syntactic Descriptions of Examined structures

The syntactic image analysis described further, aimed to understand the looked-for lesions, which are symptoms of some defined diseases, has been conducted on all examples analysed here based uniquely on the obtained width diagrams of vessels visualised on those images (following the above-described image pre-processing). To diagnose and describe the analysed lesions in the examined structures we have used context-free attributed grammars of the LR(1)-type [30]. Those grammars allow us (with an appropriate definition of primitive components) to diagnose and describe in an unambiguous way all lesions and pathological deformations important from the point of view of the diagnosis tasks analysed here. The key to success in every task performed was an appropriate definition of the primitive component set (alphabet of graph primitives), allowing to record every examined organ shape (both correct and pathologically changed) as a regular expression in the language defined by the analysed grammar. As it has already been stressed above, this task was simplified due to the fact that primitive components were defined on the vessel width diagrams obtained (as a result of pre-processing) after an execution of the straightening transformation. This did not mean, however, that indicating the necessary primitive components (and finding terminal symbols corresponding to those components) was a very easy task.

It is at the stage of selecting the primitive components that the author of the medical image understanding method described in this book must, for the first time (although not for the last time), co-operate closely with a team of experienced medical doctors. Those experienced diagnosis experts – the only competent ones – can tell which features of the analysed contour of a selected organ are connected with some stages of natural diagnostic reasoning. The role of producers of the optimum set of 'letters' of the created grammar is strictly divided: a doctor can (and should!) focus his/her attention at the largest number of details possible, treating every image discussed here as a totally new, separate case. A computer scientist must try to integrate and generalise the detailed information in such a way, that the result is a maximally compact set of primitive components as little numerous as possible; components must allow to build a computationally effective graph grammar. To some extent this work reminds of research conducted by anthropologists who work to create a system to record the speech of a tribe which does not have an alphabet yet. First all acoustic phenomena found in utterances of the tribe's members are recorded (related to articulation and co-articulation); next, a classes of similar sounds which do not differentiate between words are separated (phonemes). Finally graphic symbols (letters) are attributed to phonemes.

To use a concrete example we should state that in the tasks selected and discussed here there was a need to determine such primitive components that allowed to describe such pathological deformations, which edges of the analysed structures can undergo on the obtained width profiles. In accordance with the opinions of doctors whom we consulted, shape features important for the diagnostics are: pathological stenoses or dilations of the examined vessels and local changes of their contour such as side ramifications and cysts.

After an analysis of many examples of images it turned out that morphological lesions with very differing shapes played an identical role in the diagnostic reasoning of doctors; this resulted in that for the aggregation of those various forms of deformation of the examined vessels' contour line, it was possible to use the line approximation algorithm of the previously obtained vessel width diagram for identical sets (sequences) of primitive components. Such an approximation of the complete edge line of the diagram by means of a polygon can be a technique executed most easily by a method described in paper [31]. As a result of application of this method for every diagram, we obtain a sequence of segments approximating its external contours. This sequence simplifies the analysed image once again;

still it retains all information important from the point of view of the constructed automatic diagnostic reasoning sequence. It is worth noticing that at this stage we have a very uneven compression of the primitive image information. This is beneficial for the 'concentration of attention' of the recognising diagram operating on these contour fragments, which are really important. If a fragment of the examined vessel at some (even very long) segment of its course has a smooth form, deprived of morphological features that could be important for the recognition process, then the whole approximated segment is one section of a polygon and it will be represented by one symbol in notation based on a sequence of identifiers of the discovered graphic primitives. If, on the other hand, a contour fragment is characterised by big changes of the edge line, then the proposed form of description will attribute many segments of a polygon; this will denote its big representation in the final linguistic notification. It is rightly so since for the diagnosis this is an important fragment!

Next, depending on the parameters, the terminal symbols are attributed to each of the polygon segments. In the examples considered here, one parameter was enough to obtain a satisfactory specification of the analysed images' description; the parameter characterised every successive segment of the approximating polygon in the form of its inclination angle. To be more exact: the appropriately digitised values of the angle were given in the form of primitive components. The digitation pattern used could be treated as a counterpart of dictionary of the introduced language of shape features. Yet in more complex tasks we can imagine a situation, in which the set of primitive components can also depend on further features of the polygon approximating the examined shape, e.g. on the length of individual segments or their mutual location.

Of course, languages describing separate classes of medical images (of pancreas, heart and urinary tracts) are different. Thus concrete rules governing the creation of languages of primitive components for languages in each class are different. Formulae of concrete operations, aimed to build a specialist grammar and specialist language of description of shape features in every of the here-described cases will be presented below, while the tasks of recognition of disease types based on appropriate X-ray images are described. It will be possible to notice easily that in every case the final result of the operation is a sequence of terminal symbols, which are the input into an appropriately designed syntax analysers and syntactic transducers, the basic tool for the implementation of the process of medical image automatic understanding as described in this book.

4.4. Structural Analysis of Coronary Vessels

In this chapter we have presented methods of computer-aided diagnosis for the recognition of morphological lesions of coronary vessels with the use of syntactic methods of pattern recognition. Recognising such lesions is extremely important from the viewpoint of correct diagnosis of myocardial ischaemia states caused by coronary atheromatosis sclerosis lesions resulting in stenoses of artery lumen, which in consequence lead to myocardial ischaemia disease. This disease can take the form of either stable or unstable angina pectoris or myocardial infraction [10, 17, 22].

The objective of methods described in this chapter will be to diagnose the stenoses of coronary arteries, in particular the so-called important stenoses: artery lumen stenoses which exceed 50% and occur in the left coronary artery trunk as well as stenoses exceeding 70% of the artery lumen in the remaining segments of coronary vessels. The importance of a correct diagnosis of such lesions is demonstrated, among others, by the fact that closing the lumen of one of left coronary artery branches, e.g. interventriclar anterior artery can constitute a life threat due to the fact that it leads to ischaemia or necrosis of more than 50% of the left ventricle cardiac muscle. Examples of coronary artery images with stenoses have been shown on Figure 4.7.

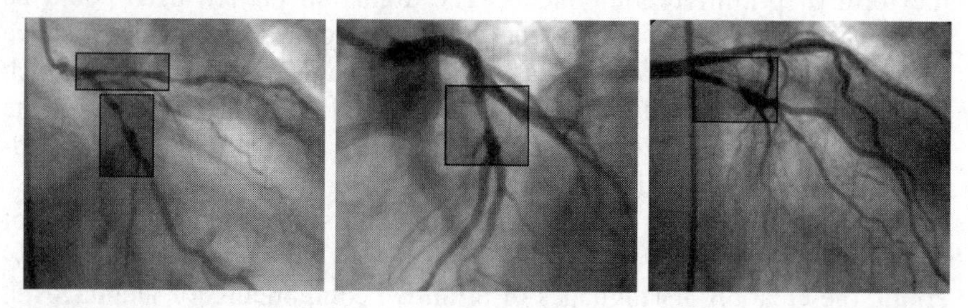

Fig. 4.7.a–c. Images of coronary arteries obtained in the course of coronography examination. The frames mark important strictures of the examined arteries, which will be localised and analysed with the use of structural pattern recognition methods

In order to diagnose correctly and to define the degree to which lesions are advanced we have proposed a context-free attributed grammar of the look-ahead LR(1) type. This grammar allows one to diagnose effectively this type of irregularities shown on X-ray images obtained in the course of coronography examinations. The main advantage of context-free grammar application, as compared to analysis methods proposed by other researchers [55], is a possibility to diagnose – on the obtained width profiles of the examined artery – both concentric strictures which in cross-sections are seen as a monotonous stenoses of the whole lumen as well as eccentric stenoses, which occur on only one vessel wall. This fact is important from the diagnostic point of view since it allows to discover if the identified symptom is characteristic for stable angina pectoris (if concentric stricture is discovered) or unstable angina pectoris (if an eccentric stenosis is discovered) [40].

Obtaining width diagrams of analysed vessels in such a way that they show both concentric and eccentric stenoses is possible owing to an application at the pre-processing stage, images of operation sequences described in the chapter devoted to medical images pre-processing, which as a result allow one to obtain width profiles of the examined structures. Figure 4.8 shows images with width profiles obtained for the first three coronary arteries presented in this chapter.

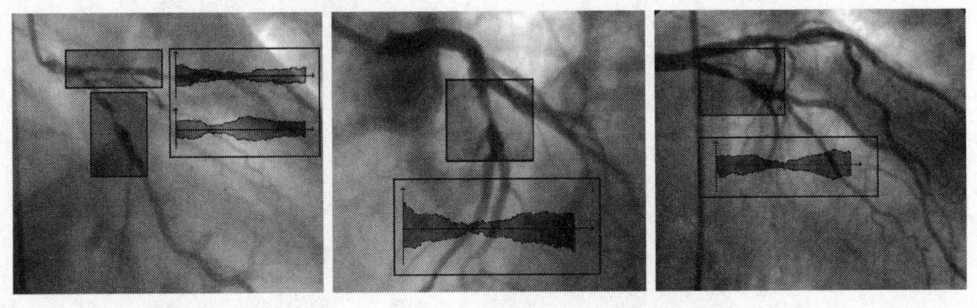

Fig. 4.8.a–c. Images of coronary arteries with visible width profiles of sections with stenoses

4.4.1 Syntactic Analysis and Diagnosing Coronary Artery Stenoses

Diagnosing looked-for morphological lesions occurring in the form of various kinds of coronary artery lumen strictures will be conducted on width diagrams obtained in the course of coronary angiogram pre-processing. Those diagrams show the width of the examined coronary vessels. To analyse them we have proposed an attributed grammar allowing the definition of all potential shapes of the expected morphological lesions.

In order to determine appropriately primitive components in the image, which will allow to create a linguistic description of the looked-for lesions, the obtained diagrams visualising coronary artery profiles undergo line approximation conducted by a method previously used by the author in comparative research [40], in the literature known as the Fast Polygonal Approximation [53]. As a result of this operation, every examined diagram obtains its own representation in the form of a sequence of approximating segments. Those segments are then attributed to successive terminal symbols forming a new linguistic representation. This representation is the input information for the syntax analyser, based on the grammar prepared and described in detail later in the book. The syntax analyser constitutes appropriate software, which will recognise all looked-for lesions of the coronary artery lumen.

The following attributed grammar has been proposed to diagnose various types of stenosis shapes:

$G_{CA} = (V_N, V_T, SP, STS)$, V_N – set of non-terminal symbols, V_T – set of terminal symbols, SP – production set, STS – grammar start symbol

V_N = {SYMPTOM, STENOSIS, H, V, NV}
V_T = {h, v, nv, λ} for h∈(-10°, 10°), v∈(11°, 90°), nv∈(-11°, -90°)
STS = SYMPTOM
SP:

1. SYMPTOM → STENOSIS   Symptom=Stenosis
2. STENOSIS → NV H V | NV V | NV H
3. V → v | V v $w_{sym} := w_{sym} + w_v$; $h_{sym} := h_{sym} + h_v$
4. NV → nv | NV nv $w_{sym} := w_{sym} + w_{nv}$; $h_{sym} := h_{sym} + h_{nv}$
5. H → h | H h $w_{sym} := w_{sym} + w_h$; $h_{sym} := h_{sym} + h_h$

In the presented grammar, the second one of the productions sequence proposed defines potential shapes of stenoses that can occur in the coronary vessel lumen. Further introductory steps in this grammar describe a linguistic formula defining the descending and ascending parts of the analysed stricture. The last production defines a horizontal segment, which can occur between those parts. Semantic variables h_e and w_e define the height and length of the terminal segment labelled *e*. Their role in diagnosing and presenting the diagnosis to doctors is auxiliary. The considerable simplicity of the grammar presented here results from a small number of morphological lesions, which this grammar describes; it proves also the significant generation power of context-free grammars applied to analyse and recognise medical images. The use of attributes is aimed to determine additional numeric parameters of the diagnosed stricture, which allow us to determine the percentage rate of the coronary artery lumen stenosis, important for the prognosis of the patient's state.

4.4.2 Recognition Results Obtained with the Use of Context-free Grammar

Owing to the application of the context-free grammar presented in the previous chapter it is possible to diagnose various types of coronary strictures with great precision. In the case of syntactic analysis with the use of those grammars we are dealing with a situation, in which the recognising software supplies, almost automatically, practically complete information about irregularities of the examined arteries.

Diagnosing irregularities occurring in the test data set has been conducted by a syntax analyser generated on the basis of a formal grammar description defined in the previous chapter. The analyser has been obtained with the use of complier of YACC grammars [16]. The notation of the grammar in the input YACC compiler grammar convention has been presented in Table 4.2. To simplify the notation and to enhance its legibility, non-semantic actions computing the height and length of the recognised symptoms have been removed.

Table 4.1 Notation of grammar recognising lesions of coronary artery morphology in the YACC compiler input convention

```
%token h v nv
%start SYMPTOM
%%
SYMPTOM    :   STENOSIS      {Symptom=Stenosis;}
STENOSIS   :   NV H V
           |   NV V
           |   NV H
           ;
     H     :   H h
           |   h
           ;
     NV    :   NV nv
           |   nv
           ;
     V     :   V v
           |   v
           ;
```

On the basis of this notation of the defined grammar, we have obtained sequences of states of the syntax analyser generated by means of the YACC compiler. This sequence forms the parser steering table used to recognise the looked-for symptoms (Table 4.3).

Table 4.2 Table of syntax analyser states for the grammar describing coronary artery lesions

```
state 0
     $accept: _SYMPTOM $end
     nv  shift 4
     .  error
     SYMPTOM  goto 1
     STENOSIS  goto 2
     NV  goto 3

state 1
     $accept: SYMPTOM_$end
     $end  accept
     .  error

state 2
     SYMPTOM:STENOSIS_     (1)
     .  reduce 1

state 3
     STENOSIS:  NV_H V
     STENOSIS:  NV_V
     STENOSIS:  NV_H
     NV :  NV_nv
     h  shift 8
     v  shift 9
     nv  shift 7
     .  error
     H  goto 5
     V  goto 6

state 4
     NV:  nv_     (8)
     .  reduce 8

state 5
     STENOSIS:  NV H_V
     STENOSIS:  NV H_     (4)
     H :  H_h
     h  shift 11
     v  shift 9
     .  reduce 4
     V  goto 10
state 6
     STENOSIS: NV V_     (3)
     V : V_v
     v  shift 12
     .  reduce 3

state 7
     NV:  NV nv_     (7)
     .  reduce 7

state 8
     H:  h_     (6)
     .  reduce 6

state 9
     V:  v_     (10)
     .  reduce 10

state 10
     STENOSIS:NV H V_     (2)
     V :  V_v
     v  shift 12
     .  reduce 2

state 11
     H:  H h_     (5)
     .  reduce 5

state 12
     V:  V v_     (9)
     .  reduce 9

5/127  terminals,  5/200  non-terminals
11/400  grammar  rules,  13/600  states
0  shift/reduce,  0  reduce/reduce conflicts reported
8/0 working sets used
memory:  states,etc.  125/0,  parser 5200/5
8/450 distinct lookahead sets
0 extra closures
8 shift entries, 1 exceptions
6 goto entries
0  entries  saved  by  goto  default
Optimizer  space  used:  input  25/0, output 5200/13
13 table entries, 0 zero
maximum  spread:  259,  maximum  offset: 259
```

In order to facilitate the interpretation of syntax analyser input states presented here, we shall explain the following:

1. Successive automate states are labelled by means of a key word '`state no`'
2. In every state in which there is an analyser, there are definitions of both actions, which a parser can perform in a given state as well as it has a description of the syntactic rule analysed in this state. Symbol '_' used in those rules is applied to specify which symbol has already been read by the analyser (symbol before the '_' sign) and in the course of the current analysis of a given rule as well as what will be the next symbol (symbol after the '_' sign).
3. In every state further parser actions are defined depending on the terminal symbol at the input. Those actions are described in the following way:

- Action of reading the input *shift* symbol recoded with sequences in the form of:

Terminal_symbol *shift* **next_state**

This means that in its current state, the analyser has a token defined by a **terminal_symbol** at its input. Therefore the analyser makes a shift locating it at the top of the stack and passes on to the next state defined by the **next_state.** As a result of this action, at the top of the stack there is the currently read terminal symbol and the current new state of the automate.

- *Reduce* action noted by a sequence in the form of:

. reduce **number_production**

This means that in the current state at the top of the stack is the right side of the production numbered **number_production.** As a result, the right side of the production is replaced by its left side. Sometimes in order to define the *reduce* action clearly, it is necessary to check the next input symbol. However, usually this reduction is performed as a default action labelled in the state table as '.'.

- Action of transition to the new state *goto* noted by a sequence in the form of:

Non-terminal_symbol *goto* **next_state**

This means that after the execution of reduction at the top of the stack there is not a **non-terminal_symbol** but the current state of the automate.

It is therefore necessary for the automate to go to a new state defined as **next_state** and to locate it at the top of the stack.

- Action of acceptance of the input sequence, *accept*. This action means that the whole input sequence has been read and that it belongs to the language generated by the grammar. This action is performed when the input symbol is the sign of the end of the input sequence ($end in the state table).
- *Error* detection action, which means that in accordance with syntactic rules the analyser cannot conduct further analysis. This situation takes place when after the read input symbol the next symbol seen cannot form with it a correct sequence describing the recognised object.

The analysing software created with the use of the YACC compiler has undergone a number of tests after its implementation. Their objective was to recognise coronary artery stenoses on a few dozen representative coronography images. Results obtained have confirmed a great usefulness of syntactic methods for diagnosing ischaemic heart disease.

The image set of test data, which has been used in order to determine in percentage figures the efficiency of a correct recognition of the size of stenoses in coronary arteries, included 55 different images obtained for patients with heart disease. In this set, we considered image sequences of patients previously analysed at the stage of the grammar construction and the recognising analyser. In order to avoid analysing identical images we selected separate images occurring a number of positions before or after the ones used originally (from DICOM sequences). The remaining images in the test data have been obtained for a new group of patients (25 persons), including five persons who have previously undergone angioplasty and in whose cases a restenosis of the previously dilated vessel has occurred. The objective of an analysis of these data was to determine in percentage the efficiency of the correct recognition of artery stenosis and to determine their size with the use of the grammar introduced. On the image data tested, the efficiency of recognition amounted to 93%. It is worth emphasising that this value refers to automatic analysis and determining the size of stenoses with the use of the procedure introduced, without a need to correct the external vessel contours manually. In this case the value of the efficiency of recognition is determined by the percentage fraction of the accurately recognised and measured vessel stenoses compared to the number of all images analysed in the test. The recognition itself meant locating and defining the type of stenosis, e.g. concentric or eccentric.

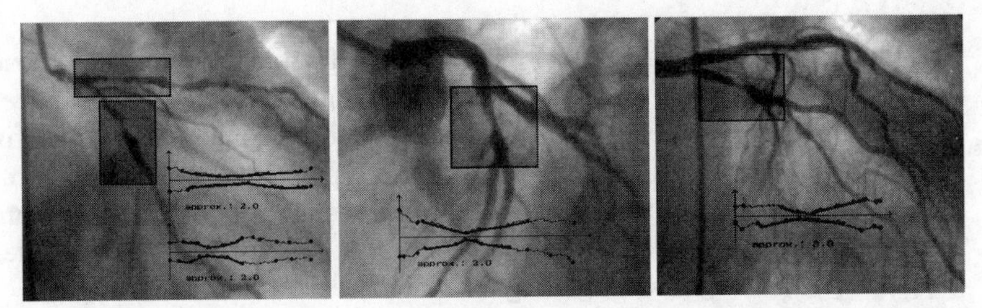

Fig. 4.9.a–c. Figures showing the result of diagnosing pathological lesions in the examined coronary arteries. The graphs visible here present width profiles of the examined arteries section with a stricture. Bold lines on diagrams mark the areas diagnosed by syntax analyser as the place where pathological strictures occur. These symptoms are of considerable diagnostic importance and they must be taken into consideration in planning further therapy

Figure 4.9 presents examples of recognising the looked-for lesions in coronary artery images analysed in this book. Recognised symptoms have been marked with a bold line.

4.4.3 Conclusion

This chapter discussed possibilities of CAD and diagnosing coronary artery lumen stenoses with the use of syntactic methods of pattern recognition. Such stenoses can be the result of the atherosclerosis lamina formation, which can lead in consequence to the development of various forms of ischaemic heart disease. This disease can be demonstrated as stable or unstable angina pectoris or as myocardial infraction. The conducted research has demonstrated that an analysis of the correct morphology of coronary artery lumen is possible owing to an application of the syntactic analysis and pattern recognition methods, in particular attributed grammars of the LR(1)-type. A deeper analysis of the results of numerous researches conducted in order to determine possibilities of diagnosing pathological lesions of coronary artery morphology have demonstrated that it is possible to apply universally the methods of mathematical linguistics to recognise and diagnose morphological lesions on medical images. Syntactic methods of pattern recognition, in particular context-free attributed grammars can constitute an additional (after their enhancement and standardisation – the basic) tool used to support early diagnosis of breast and abdominal cavity organ diseases. To this date those methods have been used – in previous works of the authors – to recognise morphological lesions in main pancreatic ducts [30] and upper urinary tracts [36]. The methodology of those tasks will be described in further chapters. Results presented in this paper demonstrate that methods described here can be also widely applied in cardiology. Possibilities of wide use of these type methods in medical image analysis result in that they can play also an important role in Picture Archiving and Communication Systems – PACS, especially as modules supporting the recognition and diagnosis of disease lesions.

4.5. Structural Analysis and Understanding of Lesions in Urinary Tract

This chapter will present the methodology of analysing and diagnosing morphological lesions occurring in upper urinary tracts. The diagnosis of these lesions has been conducted based on analysis of radiograms (urograms) of renal pelvis and upper segments of urinary tracts [35].

In the case of renal radiogram analysis, the main task is to recognise local stenoses or dilations of upper segments of urinary tracts (examples of those images have been presented on Figure 4.10) and attempt to define the correct morphology of renal pelvis and renal calyxes. Lesions in those structures can suggest the occurrence of renal calculi or deposits that by causing ureter artresia can lead to diseases such as acute extrarenal uraemia or hydronephrosis.

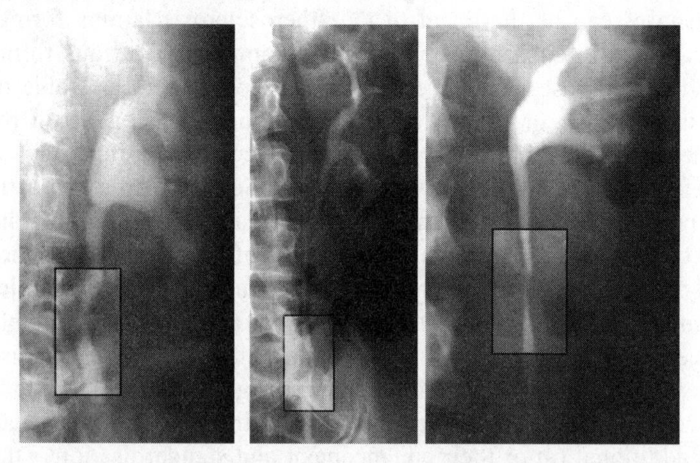

Fig. 4.10.a–c. Images obtained from urography examinations showing upper sections of the urinary tracts. Visible left renal pelvises and urinary tracts section with ureterostenosis (shown in the frames). Diagnostic analysis of this symptom will be conducted with the use of syntactic pattern recognition methods

An analysis of the correct morphology of ureter lumen will be conducted with the use of context-free attributed grammar. It is worth reminding that this type of grammars belongs to a wider class of sequential grammars [56].

The correctness analysis of renal pelvis and renal calyx will be conducted with the use of a tree grammar. Tree methods of syntactic pattern recognition are generally used to analyse more complex objects, textures or scenes in an image [56] and this is why for a nefrogram analysis they have been used to verify the correctness of the morphology of renal pelvis and renal calyx.

4.5.1 Diagnosing Stenosis of the Ureter Lumen

Diagnosing morphological lesions in the form of ureter stenosis or dilations has been conducted with the use of the following attributed grammar:

$G_U = (V_N, V_T, SP, STS)$, Where, as in the previous case V_N – stands for a set of non-terminal symbols, V_T – set of terminal symbols, SP – production set, a STS – start symbol.

V_N = {SYMPTOM, STENOSIS, DILATATION, H, V, NV}

V_T = {h, v, nv} for $h \in (-8°, 8°)$, $v \in (9°, 180°)$, $nv \in (-9°, -180°)$

STS = SYMPTOM

SP:

1. SYMPTOM → STENOSIS   Symptom=Stenosis
2. SYMPTOM → DILATATION   Symptom=Dilatation
3. STENOSIS → NV H V | NV V | NV H
4. DILATATION → V H NV | V NV | V H
5. V → v | V v $w_{sym} := w_{sym} + w_v$; $h_{sym} := h_{sym} + h_v$
6. NV → nv | NV nv $w_{sym} := w_{sym} + w_{nv}$; $h_{sym} := h_{sym} + h_{nv}$
7. H → h | H h $w_{sym} := w_{sym} + w_h$; $h_{sym} := h_{sym} + h_h$

The grammar presented here, similarly as in its counterpart used to diagnose stenoses of coronary artery lumen, is not a very complex grammar. This is due to the fact that it defines a small number of morphological lesions, which can reveal the on-going disease processes; it allows us to diagnose only various forms of stenoses and dilations characteristic for various disease units. The use of attributes also allows the determination of the numerical parameters of morphological lesions. The simplicity of grammars introduced so far results mainly from the big generation capacity of context-free grammars, understood mainly as possibilities to describe complex shapes by means of a small number of introductory rules that is grammar productions. We shall see a totally different situation in analysing and diagnosing pathological lesions in the main pancreatic ducts, where a bigger number of symptoms to be recognised and the variety of their shapes will result in that the complexity of the looked-for pathologies on the external contours can be ensured only by a more complex grammar, together with an auxiliary recognition procedure based on the use of languages of shape feature description.

4.5.2 Application of Graph Grammar in the Analysis of Renal Pelvis Shape

The analysis of the renal pelvis and the renal calyx has been accomplished with the use of G_{EDT} expansive tree grammar generating trees with directed and labelled edges, i.e. the EDT trees [56].

Although even in the right conditions, that is without visible lesions in the morphology, those structures are characterised by an extraordinary variability of shapes, it is possible to find some common features characteristic for all correct structures [18, 22]. Those features are first of all the number of smaller and bigger calyxes in the renal sinus. In correct structures there are usually only two or three bigger calyxes entering the renal pelvis; in turn those are formed by eight to ten smaller calyxes occurring in them. Smaller calyxes end with concave renal papilla forming peaks of renal pyramids, as shown on Figure 4.11.A.

Analysis of such regularities has been made with the use of an expansive tree grammar defined principally to analyse the skeleton morphology of the examined renal pelvis and renal calyx. Skeletonisation has been made with the use of the Pavlidis skeletonisation algorithm. Skeleton obtained as a result of thinning is further analysed in the following way: the first skeleton ramification point is the beginning of bigger calyxes' skeletons. Finding the number of ramifications originating in them allows us to obtain the number of larger calyxes. Determining in every bigger calyx ramifications of the next order calyx allows us to determine the number of smaller calyxes originating from it.

On the other hand, in smaller calyxes the analysis of end points in a skeleton allows us to determine if they ramify further or not. This can show if a given renal papilla is not concave towards the calyx interior but that it is convex towards the renal pyramid, as is the case with hydronephrosis or caused by cysts or in the case of neoplasm processes (Figure 4.11B). Skeletonisation of convex renal papilla leads to the formation of skeletons of those structures without further ramifications (Figure 4.11B). The result of skeletonisation of correct renal papilla, that is concave renal papilla, is skeleton lines with visible fork-like ramifications (Figure 4.11A).

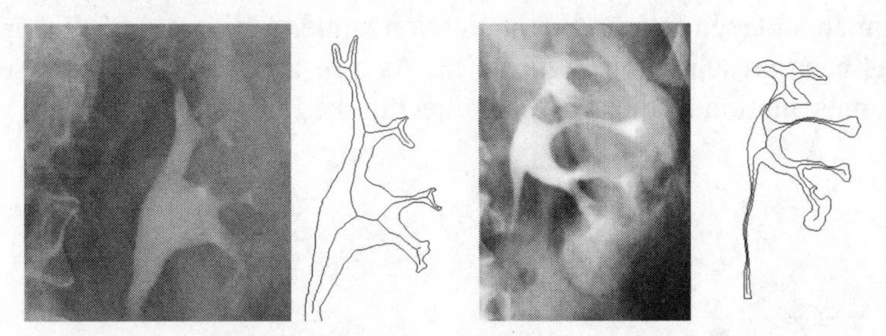

Fig. 4.11.a–b. Urograms of renal pelvis and renal calyx with skeletons obtained by means of Pavlidis skeletonisation algorithm. *a)* Correct renal pelvis, *b)* renal pelvis with symptoms of renal displasia: fibrolipomatosis

A tree grammar describing the correct skeletons of renal pelvis and renal calyx will be defined in such a way that the tree root will be defined by the location of the point where larger calyxes ramify; its successors will be determined by the ramification points of the 2nd order, that is the beginning of smaller calyxes (Figure 4.12). The last layer of peaks is defined by ramification points of the 3rd order, which is by ramifications occurring if a renal papilla has a concave shape (Figure 4.12).

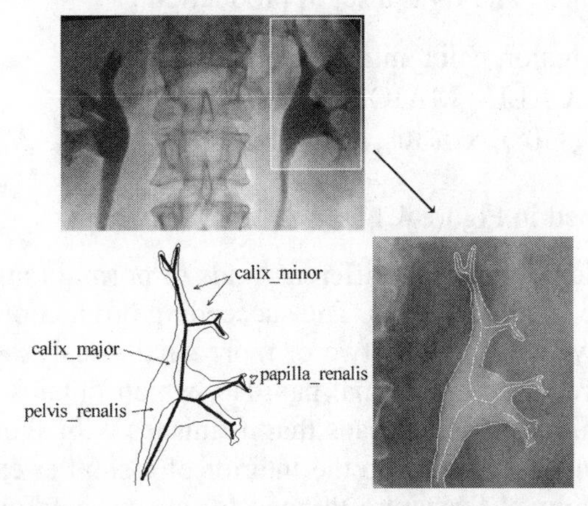

Fig. 4.12. Urogram of a healthy renal pelvis and calyxes together with the skeleton and graph description obtained after skeleton approximation

To define the primitive components used in the tree grammar we can use the approximation algorithm of skeleton ramification in renal pelvis and renal calyx. This allows us to identify every ramification with a single segment, whose ends are determined by the ends of the approximated ramification. Next, edge terminal labels are attributed to each of the determined segments, depending on the inclination angle. A diagram of this operation has been presented on Figure 4.13. As a result of the operation we obtain a representation of the analysed object in the form of a tree.

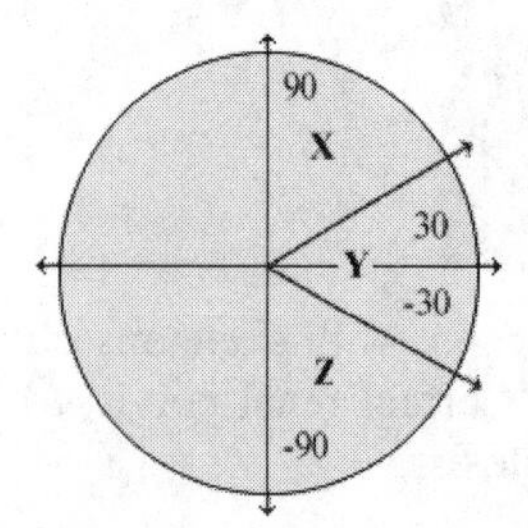

Fig. 4.13. Diagram for coding approximating segments of renal pelvis skeleton ramification into tree grammar edge labels

The following graph grammar was used to diagnose morphological changes in renal pelvises: $G_{edt}=(\Sigma, \Gamma, r, P, Z)$, where $\Sigma = \Sigma_N \cup \Sigma_T$ is a set of terminal and non-terminal vertex labels, r is a function which assigns to the graph vertex the number of its consequents, Z is a finite set of starting graphs, Γ – is a set of edge labels, and P– is a set of production.

Σ_T = {pelvis_renalis, calix_major, calix_minor, papilla_renalis}

Σ_N = {PELVIS_RENALIS, CALIX_MAJOR, CALIX_MINOR}

Γ = {x, y, z} for y∈(-30°, 30°), x∈(30°, 180°), z∈(-30°, -180°), Z = {PELVIS_RENALIS}

Set of production P is defined in Figure 4.14.

The first group of production defines the different kinds of normal renal pelvis i.e. having two or three smaller calyxes. The succeeding productions define the form of bigger calyxes formed by two or more smaller calyxes. The last group defines the proper form of renal papillae, which obtains a fork form during the skeletonisation. This means that it finishes with short branches that arise only when it is concave to the interior of a smaller calyx. During skeletonisation convex forms are thinned to the line without end branches, which results from the properties of skeletonisation algorithms.

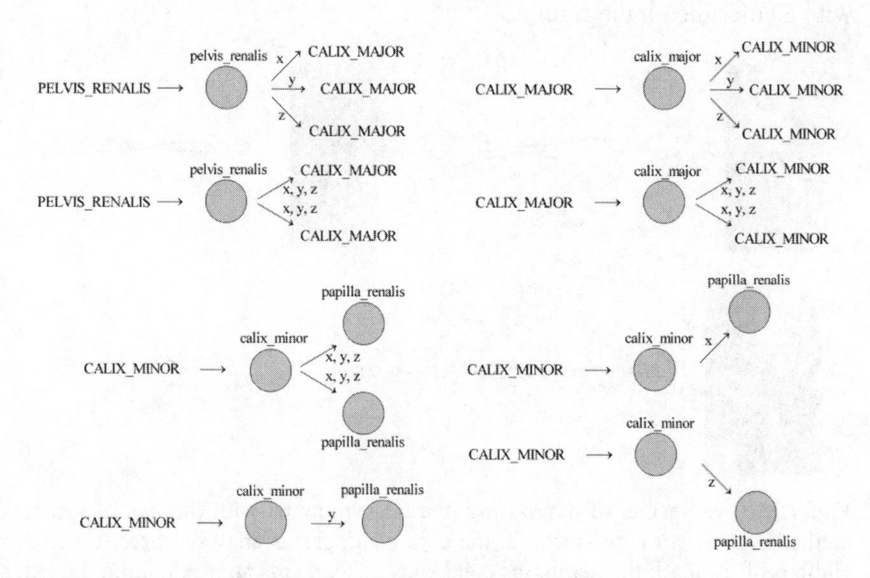

Fig. 4.14. Set of production P for the graph grammar describing the morphology of renal pelvises

The interpretation of disease lesions in the upper urinary tracts has been conducted based on a set of test images composed of 30 X-ray images showing disease lesions. These images can be divided into two groups interpreted by specialist as cases with in-born lesions and those with lesions acquired as a result of on-going disease processes (renal calculi or hydronephrosis). All of them revealed ureter lumen stenosis or anomalies in the structure of the renal sinus. The test conducted shows that the recognition efficiency of such lesions on the test data set equals about 90%. In the remaining cases interpretation difficulties resulted mainly from a change of the pathology character: from a local and distinct into a blurred lesion. The lesions in question are very large, originating as a result of neoplastic lesions, which lead to a complete change of shape or disappearance of the analysed structures. Interpretation correctness depends also on the size of the approximation threshold, which for considerably dilated ureters should be selected depending on the size of the lesion observed. Such cases often remain not fully recognised and they can diminish the whole method's efficiency.

Figure 4.15 shows examples of diagnosing the looked-for lesions in urinary tracts analysed in this chapter. The recognised symptoms are marked with a bold line on the figures.

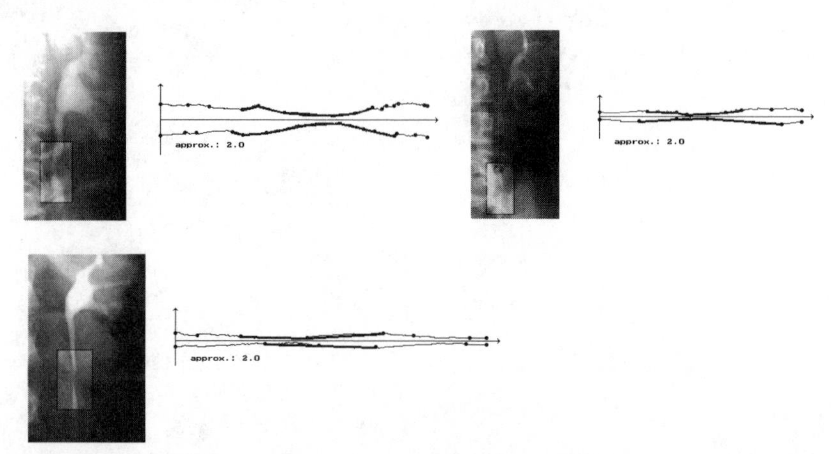

Fig. 4.15.a–c. Results of diagnosing disease symptoms with the use of syntactic methods of pattern recognition in the case of urograms analysed here. Circles on width profiles mark the beginnings and ends of segments approximating the external contour of the straightened structure

4.6. Syntactic Methods Supporting the Diagnosis of Pancreatitis and Pancreas Neoplasm

In this chapter we shall discuss possibilities to apply sequential methods of structural image analysis and understanding to morphological lesion description and to analysis of shape features of the main pancreatic ducts shown on images obtained in the course of ERCP examinations (Endoscopic Retrograde Cholangiopancreatography) [1, 30]. Those methods are aimed to determine and examine the correctness of morphological shapes of pancreatic ducts and to diagnose such pathological lesions, which demonstrate the existence of neoplasm lesions or inflammation states. Research conducted on diagnosing disease lesions in those tracts, using syntactic pattern recognition methods are also aimed to prepare algorithms and methods, which enhanced and standardised, can be used in CAD of neoplasm lesions and pancreatitis.

The objective of ERCP image analysis is to diagnose morphological lesions of pancreatic ducts characteristic for neoplasm and chronic pancreatitis. The most important symptoms characteristic for pancreas neoplasm are first of all the occurrence of local stenoses or dilations in the main pancreatic duct as well as the occurrence of cysts or cavernous projections on the external edges of the pancreatic duct (Figure 4.16.C, D). Ducts with symptoms of chronic pancreatitis can be characterised by the occurrence of irregular side ramifications of the I, II or III order as well as local stenoses or dilations (Figure 4.16.A, B). The enumerated symptoms will be recognised owing to the use of a context-free attributed grammar specially defined for this purpose, and additionally, by languages of description of shape features allowing to diagnose quickly various types of pathological convexities or stenoses.

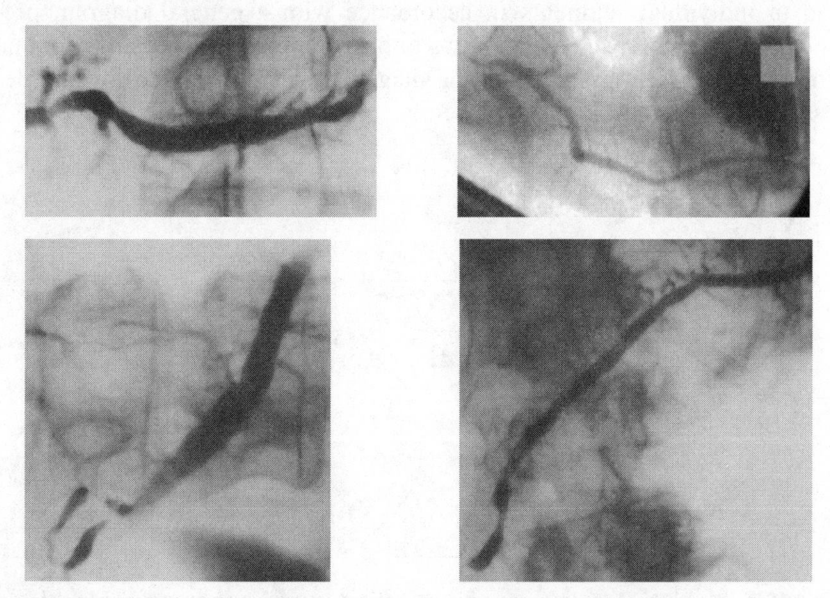

Fig. 4.16.a–d. ERCP images showing pancreatic ducts with symptoms of chronic pancreatitis and pancreas cancer

The analysis of the looked-for morphological lesions has been conducted based on width diagrams obtained during image pre-processing, with the use of context-free attributed grammars of the LR(1)-type. Such grammars, similarly as in the previous tasks, with the appropriate definition of primitive components on width diagrams and primitive terminal symbols corresponding to those, allow us to diagnose – on ERCP images – all pathological lesions important from the diagnostic point of view: cysts, strictures, dilations and ramifications.

The use of attributes in this grammar allows, similarly as it did earlier, to determine additional information defining the width and height of the discovered pathology; this can be used for diagnosing numerous uncertain or ambiguous cases.

In order to determine primitive components, which will allow to describe entirely on the obtained width profiles the edges of pancreatic ducts, we have used the previously applied algorithm of line approximation for diagrams with the Fast Polygonal Approximation method. As a result, for each diagram we obtain a sequence of its segments approximating it (Figure 4.17.a).

Next, depending on the angle of inclination, terminal symbols are attributed to individual segments in accordance with a general diagram presented on Figure 4.17.b. This allows to obtain input sequences of terminal symbols for parsers recognising the diagnostic lesions looked-for and defined by the grammar introduced below.

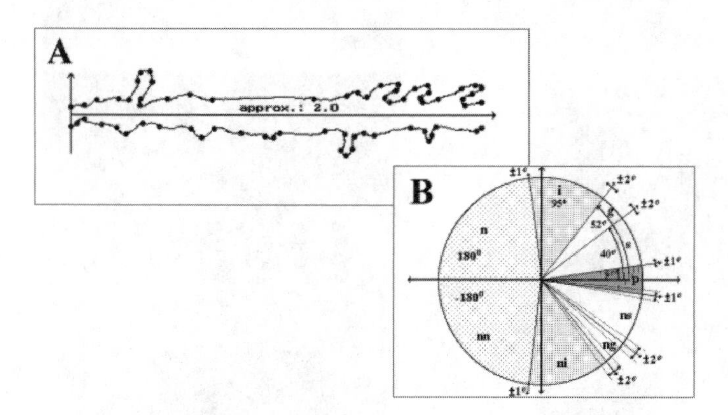

Fig.4.17.a. Width profile diagram of pancreatic duct with symptoms of chronic inflammation; marked segments have been obtained as a result of its approximation with accuracy $\varepsilon=2$. **b**. The diagram shows coding segments approximating diagrams of pancreatic ducts into terminal symbols

4.6.1 Context-free Grammar in the Analysis of Shapes of Pancreatic Ducts

The following attributed grammar has been used to describe morphological lesions in the examined pancreatic ducts: $G = (V_N, V_T, SP, STS)$, where

V_N = {LESION, CYST, STENOSIS, DILATATION, BRANCH, P, S, G, I, N, NS, NG, NI, NN}

V_T = {p, s, ns, g, ng, i, ni, n, nn}, where p∈(-9°, 9°), s∈(9°, 40°), ns∈(-9°, -40°), g∈(40°, 52°), ng∈(-40°, -52°), i∈(52°, 95°), ni∈(-52°, -95°), n∈(95°, 180°), nn∈(-95°, -180°),

STS = LESION

SP:

1. LESION → CYST | STENOSIS Lesion=Cyst; Lesion=Stenosis
2. LESION → DILATATION | BRANCH Lesion=Dilatation; Lesion=Branch
3. CYST → I P NI | G P NG | I P NG | G P NI | I S NI | G S NG | I S NG | G S NI | I NS NI | G NS NG | I NS NG | G NS NI
4. STENOSIS → NS S | NS G | NS P S | NS P I | NG S | NI NS I | NI S
5. DILATATION → S P NG | S G NS | S NS | G NS
6. BRANCH → I NI | I NS | I P NI NN | I NS NI NN | G NI | G S NN | G P NN | G S NI NN | S NG | S NS NN | N G NG NI
7. N → n | N n $\{w_{sym} = w_{sym} + w_n;\ h_{sym} = h_{sym} + h_n\}$
8. NN → nn | NN nn $\{w_{sym} = w_{sym} + w_{nn};\ h_{sym} = h_{sym} + h_{nn}\}$
9. I → i | I i $\{w_{sym} = w_{sym} + w_i;\ h_{sym} = h_{sym} + h_i\}$
10. NI → ni | NI ni $\{w_{sym} = w_{sym} + w_{ni}\}$
11. G → g | G g $\{w_{sym} = w_{sym} + w_g;\ h_{sym} = h_{sym} + h_g\}$
12. NG → ng | NG ng $\{w_{sym} = w_{sym} + w_{ng}\}$
13. S → s | S s $\{w_{sym} = w_{sym} + w_s;\ h_{sym} = h_{sym} + h_s\}$
14. NS → ns | NS ns $\{w_{sym} = w_{sym} + w_{ns}\}$
15. P → p $\{w_{sym} = w_{sym} + w_p;\ h_{sym} = h_{sym} + h_p\}$

Semantic rules of the first productions specify the type of the looked-for disease lesion while productions define the basic types of such diseases. Further productions define possible shapes of such pathologies. The last group specifies the shapes of descending and ascending arms in the morphology of such disease symptoms. Semantic variables of those productions allow specifying numerical parameters of the recognised lesion.

4.6.2 Languages of Shape Feature Description in the Analysis of Pancreatic Duct Morphology

For a correct description and recognition of symptoms, for which a 2D analysis is necessary on the obtained width diagrams (that is, for example, big cavernous projections), additional languages of description of shape features with multi-directional sin quad distribution [24, 28] have been used. Those languages have also been used due to an impossibility to define precisely all potential shapes that the looked-for lesions can take. The main advantage of these languages is that the recognition process can be based on an analysis of features describing the essence of those shapes, that is the occurrence of lesions such as, for example, concavities or dilations. Those languages, owing to an application of a sequential transducer with multiple inputs allow the recognition of some lesions without the need to define their morphology precisely but only based on transitions between the so-called sinquads (that is specified directions of the sectors approximating the width diagrams). Intervals determining the directions of the basic sin quads in an analysis of pancreatic ducts have been shown on Figure 4.18. This analysis is more universal in its character than the analysis with the use of grammars. This is due to the fact that it enables an identification of all types of convexities, ramifications and stenoses – even in situations in which those lesions are not recognised by the previously described context-free grammar.

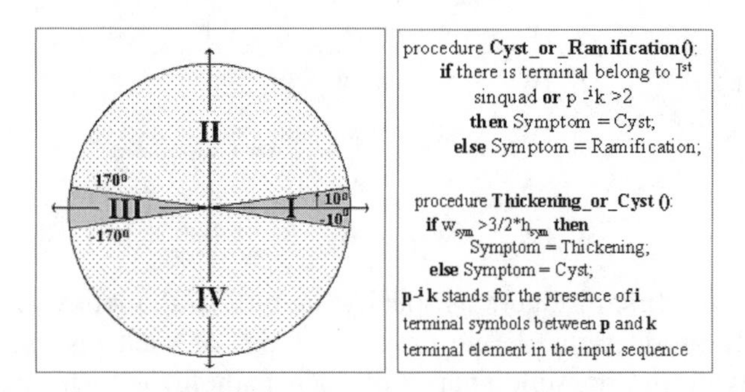

Fig. 4.18. Diagram showing the sin quad distribution for the analysis of morphological lesions together with semantic procedures recognising cysts, ramifications and dilations

The representation of the looked-for lesions with the use of the method based on defining spatial directions presented on Figure 4.18 is extremely simple. Direction I determine the location of those segments in the pancreatic duct, which do not have pathological morphological lesions (similarly as interval III in the case of analysis beginning with the end of the duct). The remaining intervals determine the directions of segments approximating the external contours of those duct parts, in which lesions have occurred. A detection of a given lesion is possible owing to an analysis of transitions between individual sin quads. In Table 4.4 we defined the main transitions between various sin quads corresponding to individual disease symptoms.

Table 4.3. Transitions between sin quads characterising individual disease symptoms

Symptom	Sin quad transition
Side ramification	II → IV
Cysts and dilations	II → IV or II → I → IV (in reverse analysis also II → III → IV)
Stenoses	IV → II and IV → I → II (or IV → III → II)

Due to the fact that the transitions given here do not specify in an unambiguous way lesions, to identify them accurately it is necessary to use the previously defined attributes of those symptoms and to conduct the following semantic procedures allowing to differentiate between a cyst and a side ramification as well as between a cyst and a local dilation in the main pancreatic duct:

Procedures `Cyst_or_Ramification()` and `Thickening_or_Cyst()` are executed at the moment when the syntax analyser recognises a cyst, ramification or dilation. Those procedures are supposed to confirm the correctness of ambiguous case recognition. In a production set describing cyst features there are introductory rules which allow us also to describe the external contours of small ramifications (e.g. lack of horizontal section and acute inclination angles of the approximating segment). Also high and short dilations in the duct can, as a matter of fact, turn out to be cysts.

Conditions defining the procedure

```
Cyst_or_Ramification():
if (terminal belonging to I sinquad occurred
         or
 p-k^i > 2) then Symptom=Cyst;
                              Else Symptom = Ramification;
```

Where symbol $p \overset{i}{-} k$ stands for the occurrence of elements (terminal symbols) between the initial (p) and final (k) terminal element from the input symbol recognised by the analyser as sequence defining the pathological pattern.

Those conditions mean that if, during the syntactic analysis of the input sequence of terminal symbols, in a correctly recognised sequence describing one of pathologies, a terminal belonging to sin quad I appears (that is one defining the horizontal component of this representation), than the recognised symptom is a classic cyst. Similarly, in the case in which the analyser classifies a larger number of terminal symbols in the course of recognition, also then the recognised element is a cyst; this is due to the fact that the property of ramifications is their simple form, usually described by two terminal symbols of which the first one describes the ascending arm while the other one the descending arm on width profile diagrams.

Conditions defining the procedure

```
Thickening_or_Cyst ():
          if (wsym >3/2*hsym ) then Symptom =
Thickening;
           else Symptom = Cyst;
```

where w_{sym}, h_{sym} – respectively stand for the length and height of the pathological symptom, as determined on the width profile of the analysed pancreatic duct.

This condition means that if a discovered anomaly has its width by half bigger than its height, then this symptom should be classified as a local dilation. In the other case we are dealing with a cyst. This condition is based on an assumption that a cyst has a shape which is more convex than wide.

4.6.3 Results of Syntactic Method Analysis of Pancreatic Ducts

Despite the complicated grammatical reasoning process, also in this case the syntactic methods of pattern recognition supply practically all information on morphological lesions on the external edges of the pancreatic ducts analysed here.

Similarly as it is for grammars analysing coronary arteries and ureteres, also in this case – for the sequential grammar presented in this chapter, a syntax analyser has been constructed in the form of a parser generated with the use of the YACC compiler. This analyser has been subject to a number of experiments. As a result it obtained very good results in recognising the looked-for lesions on ERCP images. In the case of analysis of those images, additionally a sequential transducer has been implemented for the shape feature analysis procedure, a counterpart of syntax analyser for languages of shape feature description.

This transducer, in accordance with definition, has been defined in the following way:

$ST = (Q, \Sigma_T, \Delta, \delta, Q_0)$, where Q – finite set of states, Σ_T – finite set of input (terminal) symbols, Δ – finite set of output symbols, Q_0 – set of initial states, δ – transition function defined as: $\delta : Qx\Sigma^*{}_T \longrightarrow Qx\Delta^*$.

In our case the individual sets and transition function have been defined in the following way:

$Q = \{q_1, q_2, q_3, q_4\}$ – set of transducer states

$\Sigma_T = \{ s_{ij}, i=1,3,5,7; j=1, 2, 3, 4 \}$, i – defines the component type and *j* – the sinquad number

$\Delta = \{ 1, 2, 3, 4\}$ – set of input symbols = sinquad numbers

$Q_0 = \{q_1, q_2, q_3, q_4\}$ – set of initial states

δ – transition function defined on Figure 4.19.

Sequential Multiply Entry Transducer

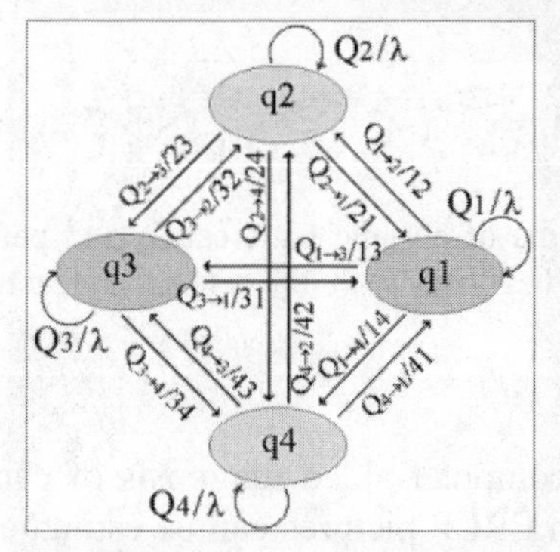

qi – denotes the ith state of transducer, i=1,2,3,4 – number of sinquad

Qi /λ – denotes that in the ith state appear terminal belonging to i^th sinquad and no symbol is writing to output (λ – an empty symbol)

Qi → j/ij - denotes that in the ith state appear terminal belonging to j^th sinquad and sequence "ij" is writing to output

Fig. 4.19. Sequential transducer with multiple input. qi stands for the ith state of the transducer, and j for the number of the analysed sinquad

On this diagram every edge connecting state qi with qj and marked with a label stands for:

1. $Q_{i \to j} / ij$ means that in the q_i state a component occurred, which belonged to the jth sinquad. A transition to state q_j occurs and the 'ij' sequence is written to the output.
2. Q_i / λ means that in the q_i state a component occurred which belonged also the ith sinquad and nothing is written to the output.

The transducer presented in this diagram supported the process of disease symptom recognition. The recognition of lesions in pancreatic ducts has been conducted based on a set of a few dozen pancreatograms including images with symptoms of chronic pancreatitis and pancreas neoplasm. The overall test set of pancreatograms available included over 100 images of neoplasm and chronic pancreatitis as well as images with healthy pancreatic ducts.

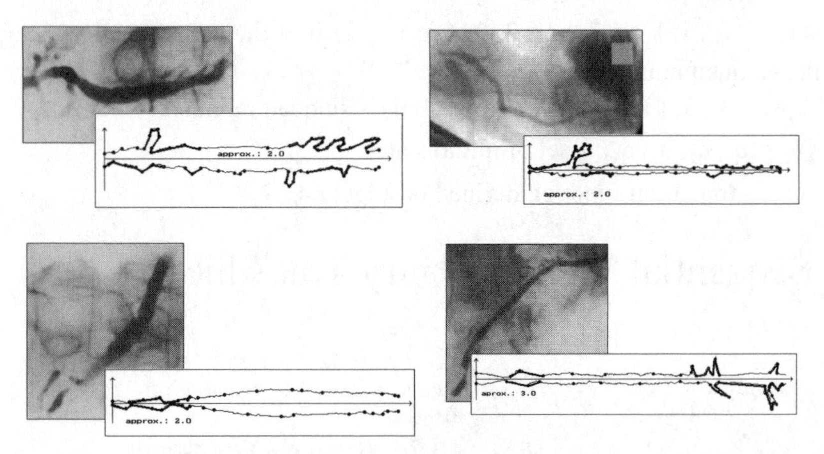

Fig. 4.20.a–d. Pancreatic ducts with symptoms of chronic pancreatitis and pancreas cancer. Result of disease symptoms diagnosis with the use of syntactic methods

The effectiveness of this methods in computer-aided diagnosis of cancerous and inflammatory lesions based on ERCP pictures can be estimated at 90%. This value stands for the percentage of correct recognitions of symptoms defined in the grammar: symptoms in the form of strictures, ramifications and lesions with cyst-like features. The remaining 10 percent of the analysed pancreas images, which were not fully correctly interpreted, can be considered to be cases difficult to interpret. Such images can present, among others, incorrect ramifications looping on the main image with the pancreatic duct or show amputation (discontinuation) of the duct. Recognition of these may require either 3D analysis or independent interpretation of separated duct parts. Some images, similarly as in the case of artery and ureter images, should be analysed with a dynamically selected approximation threshold. These cases are also included into the group of images difficult for interpretation.

Figures 4.20 present examples of recognition of looked-for lesion in ERCP images discussed above. The recognised symptoms have been marked with a thick line.

4.7. Analyses of MR images of spinal cord

Another interesting application of syntactic approach to automatic perception analysis is a morphological classification of spinal cord diseases and the diseases of surrounding spinal meninges. This chapter will show an exemplary analysis of such structures based on an examination of congenital and acquired lesions in the cord structure, visible on images obtained in the magnetic resonance technique (MR).

Among the defects of the central nervous system, including the spinal cord, there are many various types of diseases of different aetiology. These can be congenital or acquired defects manifested in the form of some concrete lesions in various spinal cord sections or in the form of nervous system dysfunctions. Apart from typical spinal cord diseases, there are also cerebrospinal meningitis states caused by the intrusion of bacteria, viruses or other parasites into the central nervous system. Inflammatory conditions can affect the white or the grey matter or the whole cord width; they can they take the form of either diffused, disseminated or focal inflammation. It is these very serious cases that can be subjected to semantic analysis by structural classifiers. Diffuse diseases of the spinal cord can be caused also by lesions in anterior and posterior spinal arteries, whose occlusion can aggravate significantly the patient's condition and lead to dangerous paralyses, sometimes even paralysis of all limbs. Spinal cord damages of vascular origin are the consequence of rupture, thrombus or embolism of such a vessel.

Apart from diseases caused by blood vessel diseases, there are also spinal cord tumours and spinal canal tumours. Spinal cord tumours can originate from the spinal cord tissue, sensory roots of the spinal nerve, meninges or the spinal cord vascular rete, the vertebrae and sometimes also from organs in the direct vicinity of disks. There can also be metastases from other body parts.

In the case of analysis of backbone and spinal cord MRI images, the chief objective in the recognition is to detect and diagnose lesions that might evidence a whole range of various disease units: from myelomeningocele, numerous forms of inflammatory conditions or cerebral or spinal cord ischaemia, to most serious cases of intra- and extradullary tumours. An unambiguous identification of all units with the use of one recognising software is extremely difficult due to rather subtle differences, critical to the correct classification of every one of them. All the same, structural analysis proves to be extremely useful in the specification of the degree of the disease unit development by means of specifying the size of lesions in the cord morphology and by defining the compression of the spinal cord and meninges [22].

The analysis of this structure uses a developed context-free grammar. It allows us to identify symptoms and to draw diagnostic conclusions relating to the inner nature of the visible pathology.

The grammar developed for the analysis of spinal cord images is defined as follows: Gsc=(Vn, Vt, STS, SP), where

Vn = {LESION, NARROWING, ENLARGEMENT, H, E, N}
Vt = {h, e, n} for $h \in [-11°, 11°]$, $e \in (11°, 180°)$, $n \in (-11°, -180°)$
STS = LESION
SP:

1. LESION → ENLARGEMENT   Lesion=enlargement
2. LESION → NARROWING   Lesion=narrowing
3. ENLARGEMENT → E H N | E N | E H
4. NARROWING → N H E | N E | N H
5. H → h | h H $w_{sym}:=w_{sym}+w_h$; $h_{sym}:=h_{sym}+h_h$
6. E → e | e E   ...
7. N → n | n N   ...

This grammar permits us to detect different forms of stenoses and dilations which may characterize the different disease units (for example neoplasm or inflammation processes).

Fig 4.21 shows an example of the spinal cord image subject to analysis. The spinal cord, after the threshold operation, is shown in Fig 4.22.

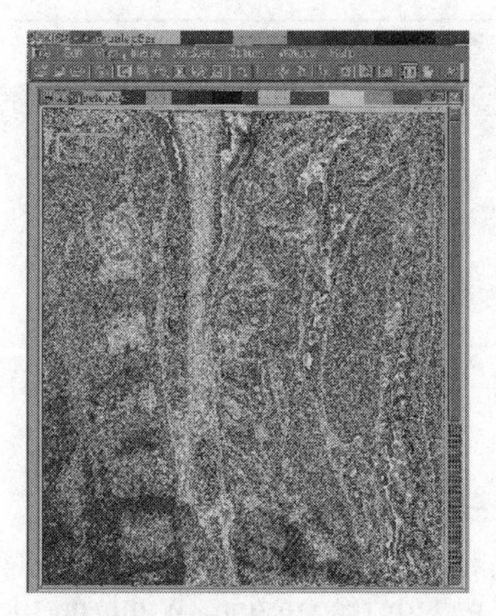

Fig. 4.21. Image of a spinal cord. The arrow indicates a lesion

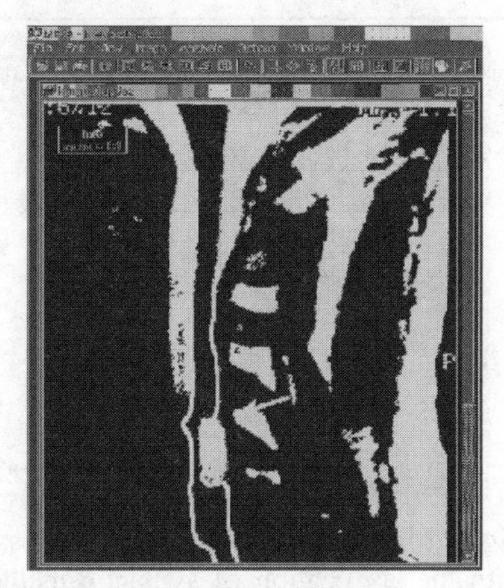

Fig. 4.22. Spinal cord image after binary conversion

The results of spinal cord morphology analysis aimed at locating pathological lesions are provided in Fig. 4.23.

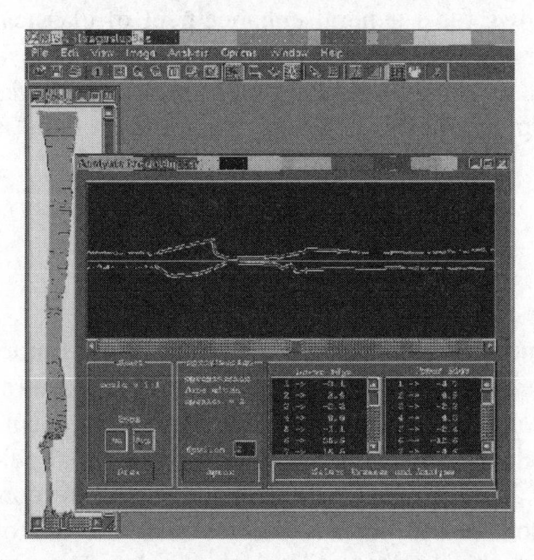

Fig. 4.23. Diagram of a spinal cord. The red colour indicates the occurrence of pathologies in the spinal cord

Another example of MR image; visible compression on the spinal cord is shown in Fig.4.24.

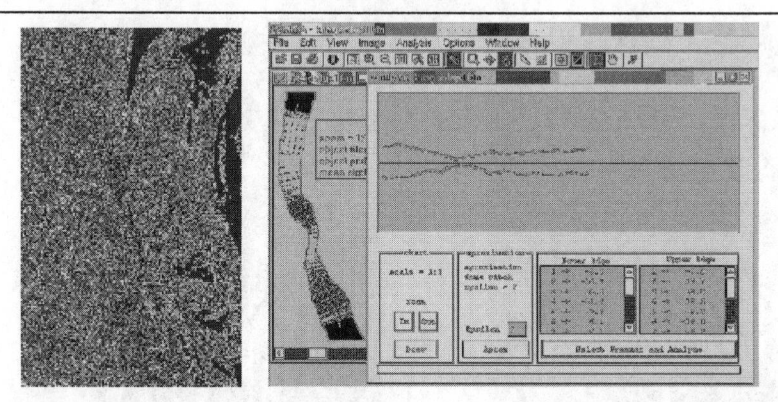

Fig. 4.24.a–b. The results of the disease symptom recognition and understanding with the application of syntactic methods of pattern recognition. Width profiles indicate the spots where the looked-for lesion was diagnosed. On the left, the original image showing spinal cord with disk herniation. On the right, the recognised place with compression of the thecal sac

As you can see, the method of cognitive medical image analysis described in the introduction allows for a general enhancement of classical image recognition methods targeted at deeper image interpretation. As it was mentioned in the previous sections, there is a great number of images that can be automatically interpreted in this manner. Among them there is also a class of images showing lesions in the central nervous system.

4.8. Results

This chapter has presented a specialist analysis and understanding of morphological shapes of selected organs of abdominal cavity, chest and central nervous system conducted in order to diagnose disease symptoms occurring in the main pancreatic ducts, upper segments of ureters and renal pelvis as well as coronary arteries and the spinal cord. The analysis of the correct morphology of these structures has been conducted with the use of sequential and graph methods belonging to syntactic methods of pattern recognition.

Owing to the application of the presented context-free grammars, it is possible to detect quite precisely the different kinds of irregularities in investigated structures.

The results of the analyses obtained until now, made on representative images, are very promising and forecast significant efficiency in the analysis of a large group of test data.

The presented methods of syntactic description are basically an attempt at automating a specifically human process of understanding what is the medical meaning of various organ shapes on a digital image; they are not just an attempt at simple recognition. In particular, a diagnosis may result from an automatic shape understanding; it is also possible to draw other numerous medical conclusions. Information can suggest a method of treatment, that is different types of therapy may be recommended, depending on the shape and pathological location described in the grammar.

Results obtained owing to the application of the above-characterised methods confirm the immense usefulness of syntactic methods in diagnosing cardiac ischemic diseases, urinary tract disabilities and inflammation as well as pancreas neoplasm processes.

4.9. Conclusions

The research carried out by the authors into the possibilities of recognising pathological changes in the morphology of coronary arteries and renal pelvises, along with upper parts of the ureter and spine have confirmed the universality of the application of the mathematical linguistic method for the recognition and analysis of morphological changes in medical images. Syntactical methods of pattern recognition and, in particular, the attributed context-free grammars, can be an additional tool supporting early diagnosis of chest organ and abdominal cavity diseases. The great efficiency of the presented algorithms makes these methods an unusually useful tool from a practical point of view in the domain of scientific engineering; they allow us to enhance and recognise essential diagnostic features in the analysis of medical images.

This chapter proves that the presented methods have an application in cardiology and nephrology as well as in endoscopy examinations. However, due to the small amount of test data, the improvement of these methods is an on-going process while the necessity of further research relates mainly to the recognition of renal pelvis pathologies with the use of graph grammar analysis. To date, the results of such analyses undertaken on several dozen representative images are very promising, and suggest a high efficiency of recognition in the analysis of a large amount of test data.

Syntactic methods of pattern recognition presented in this paper have an enormous application in the field of artificial intelligence and medical IT, especially in the field of computer medical imaging and computer-aided diagnosis (CAD). Those methods, originating from mathematical linguistics allow not only diagnosing and creating formal and advanced descriptions for complicated shapes of disease symptoms carrying diagnostic information. They can also be used to create intelligent computer systems constructed for the purpose of image perception: allowing us to obtain a definition and machine-interpretation of semantic contents of the examined image. Those systems may assist the operation of medical robots widely used in operational theatres of various surgeries. They can constitute also an integral part of CAD systems or intelligent information systems managing pictorial medical data bases located (scattered) in various places.

5. The application of the Image Understanding Technology to Semantic Organisation and Content-Based Searching in Multimedia Medical Data Bases

In recent years the knowledge of engineering has become one of the most dynamically developing branches of intelligent IT systems, including the PACS, Computer-Aided Diagnosis and medical data bases. Specialist medical data bases storing data in visual form constitute a large group of multimedia data bases; those patterns originate from numerous diagnostic examinations of practically all organs of the human body. One of the main problems with accessing and analysing information collected in this way is how to transform efficiently the visual information transfer of those patterns into a form enabling intelligent analysis and understanding of medical meaning of these patterns.

One of basic problems in accessing and fast search for useful information in multimedia data bases is the creation of a method of representation and indexing important objects constituting data contents. The task of semantic search for useful information (i.e. relating to the content, not the form of data) was discussed a number of times and to some degree it is solved for data bases including texts exclusively. Unfortunately, the introduction of multimedia data bases has demonstrated once again that the search for useful information on the basis of their content is a problem to which a practical solution is still impossible to find. Everything seems to suggest that techniques of syntactic pattern analysis, useful in computer-aided medical diagnosis, can prove very useful in the tasks of automatic search of visual data in multimedia data bases.

One of the main problems in accessing information collected in medical data bases is the way in which to transform efficiently the visual information transfer of patterns into a form enabling intelligent selection of cases obtained as an answer to queries directed at selected elements of contents of the searched-for images. Therefore this chapter will present the possibilities of application of grammars presented earlier, used as the ordering factor indexing and supporting commitment and semantically-oriented search for visual information in multimedia medical data bases.

It is worthwhile to pay attention to the essence of the semantic analysis which allows for content-based grouping of images, sometimes completely different in form, however, conveying similar diagnostic information about the disease process. Generally speaking, this is connected with a great variety of the examined cases.

In such images a concrete shape of incorrectness can vary between cases due to the fact that organs of individual people differ in shape, size and location while forms taken on by pathological lesions (e.g. caused by neoplasm or chronic inflammation process) are also unforeseeable in their details. On the other hand, every type of disease leads to some characteristic types of changes in the shapes of visualised organs; therefore this very type of information, obtained owing to the application of the structural pattern analysis method, will constitute information label determining the content of the image. Techniques proposed in this book allow the changing of a pattern into its syntactic description in such a way that the automatically generated language formula transforms precisely the basic pattern content: the shape of the examined organ and its incorrectness caused by disease. Those formalised, automatically generated descriptions of objects shapes seen on a pattern placed or searched-for in a data base, allow separating the indexation process from secondary formal features of the recorded patterns. Description is focused on the most important contents.

The idea presented here and relating to creating indexing keys allows for an efficient image search and categorisation – in the framework of one data base – both of information specifying the type of medical imaging or the examined structure as well as the meaningful semantic information specifying the looked-for object. In a special case, apart from the main indexing key allowing to search or archive a concrete type of medical images (ERCP, urograms, coronograms or spinal cord images), it is possible to create additional indexing labels specifying successive layers of semantic details of image contents. The said information is first of all the degree to which a given disease is advanced (e.g. neoplasm lesions or inflammation) detected with the use of the above-described grammars and semantic actions defined in them. The indexing information is also a description of the external morphology of the organ analysed on the image. This type of description takes the form of a terminal symbol sequence introduced while grammars are defined for individual types of images and organs visible on them. The shape morphology described in this way requires a much smaller memory and computation input for the execution of the archiving operations and for searching for a given pattern. Finally, the lowest level of information useful for a detailed search are the types of lesions recognised (irregular ramifications or stenoses etc.) and sequences of production numbers leading to a generation of a linguistic description of those lesions. Such productions are defined in the sequential and graph grammars introduced in previous chapters. Their sequences describe successive patterns of morphological lesions and can constitute important information useful for a quick search for such irregularities on image data. In the case in which graph grammars are applied – their application shall be demonstrated on the example of a description of important morphology shape features for the structure of the renal sinus (renal pelvis and renal calyx); the idea of application of the description created in this way is analogous. This grammar allows us to create an indexing key specifying – apart from the general diagnostic assessment – the number of smaller and bigger calyxes occurring in a renal pelvis. The general structure of semantic information and indexing keys has been presented on Figure 5.1.

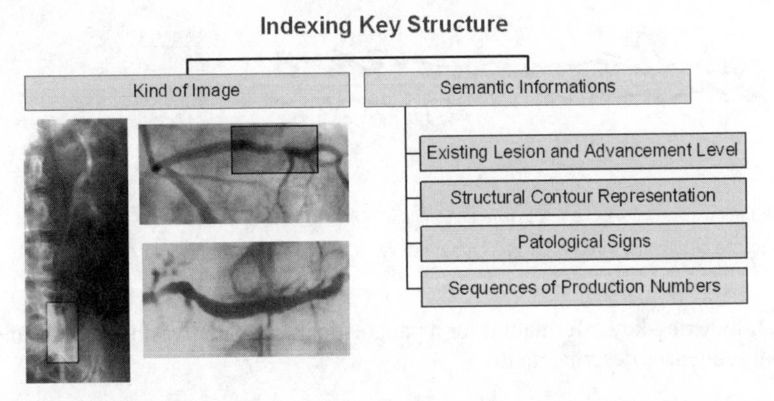

Fig. 5.1. A general scheme of semantic information and indexing key structure

The semantic approach to indexing and searching of multimedia medical data bases seems to be a more efficient and appropriate method than the traditional indexing methods [2, 19, 23] due to the presence of distinguishable objects visible in the discussed medical patterns, which by virtue of their shape define pathological disease symptoms. A structural description of medical image contents becomes easier and more unambiguous than an analogous description applied to a different category of patterns (for example scenes). Nevertheless, after defining an appropriate graph grammar, the methodology described here can be utilised to describe any pattern. It will therefore enable the creation of object-oriented semantic description of contents of those data and it will also constitute the key to their indexation and search. An additional advantage of structural description methods is a potential of additional analysis of the examined images in the course of archiving and defining the semantic meaning of lesions visible on them; this is performed by imitating a qualified professional's understanding of medical images.

Syntactic information, together with contour representation in the form of terminal symbols as well as production number sequences describing the discovered pathologies constitute the representation of patterns placed in the data base or searched-for. An example of information constituting such indexing key for a pancreatic duct image is presented in Figure 5.2.

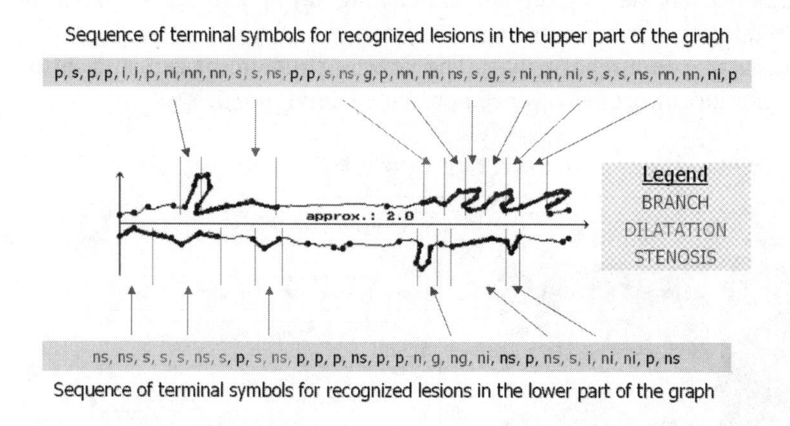

Fig. 5.2. Indexing key information for a pancreatic duct image. Visible lesions and terminal sequences describe them

In the course of selected image analysis in each case we obtain a type of recognised symptom and a sequence of production numbers, which lead to grammar derivation of shape description of such lesions. Such sequences create the proper description of analysed shapes and are stored in indexing record. In every case those spots are highlighted there, where irregularities have been identified. For each of them there are detailed descriptions in the software representation relating to the previously listed information used as indexing keys. In the case of a pancreatic duct image, the said information is presented in more detail on the image shown in Figure 5.2.

The approach to the generation of structural-semantic representation of medical patterns in multimedia data bases with the use of context-free and EDT graph grammars presented in this study is an entirely new solution.

Preliminary research reveals that such approach proves to be an extremely efficient and universal tool enabling visual data compression and unambiguous data representation. An important point is that the proposed indexation technique has been optimised with an aim to find diagnostic information, easily observed in the shape of organs visible on patterns and dependent on disease symptoms.

The main strength of the proposed structural methods for indexation and search for data in medical visual data bases is its high efficiency due to small memory complexity of semantic representation generated to represent patterns; besides algorithms used to search for similar patterns are not time-consuming. Accordingly, such search boils down to comparing the sequences of symbols representing the semantic content of analysed images, involving the search for the descriptions most similar to that of a given object in data base (it is done as visual query). This type of search operations are unaffected by minor disturbances (noise) or geometrical transformations of patterns as these factors are independent of the generated syntactic and semantic representation.

In the presented examples of coronography, urogram patterns and pancreas visualisation, a semantic descriptor created by the described methodology allows the diagnosis of a disease on the basis of a single pattern; it serves also as a key for indexation in searching for data in the data base. Those properties result from the unambiguity of representation generated for various semantic contents.

In practical terms the result of computer implementation of the syntactic analysis algorithms provided here is a developed system allowing for structural analysis of the discussed medical patterns targeted at creation of semantic representation defining various disease symptoms. The research confirmed the highest potential of developing the description of visible deformations of shapes as well as semantic categorisation of various disease symptoms. Those descriptions can be used as results of important lesions recognition. Yet, from the point of view of knowledge engineering, they may also serve as data for deeper reasoning and be used by CAD systems (Computer-Aided Diagnosis).

6. Strengths and Weaknesses of the Image Understanding Technology Compared to Previously Known Approaches

The techniques of automatic image understanding, presented in this book, utilising the linguistic approach have several major advantages over classical image recognition algorithms. It is readily apparent that for many types of images, in particular medical images, it is difficult to interpret and define the representative vector of numerical features required in the classical approach applied in theoretical decision-based methods. This means that a certain type of images containing structural information can be extremely difficult or even impossible to classify on the basis of selected features represented in numerical form. This is so because the structures ought to be described in such a manner that some relationships and constituent elements of the structure are first defined while the structure itself can be described in general terms with a use of a model or strictly specified. The presence of semantic information requires therefore that analysis be made, both of the classification and description (meaning) sense. The classification task is based chiefly on operations of seeking similarities (usually referred to as the grammar derivation path); yet this operation has some generalisation properties and together with semantic information obtained in the course of analysis, it allows us to recognise a practically unlimited number of classes and objects. An interesting point is that potentially identical objects, included to same class on account of their geometry, are owing to semantic information be distinguished and they can even constitute very distant classes of patterns. Examples of such images can easily be shown during the analysis of pancreas radiograms discussed in this book. The feature of generalisation and semantic diversification are the most important elements making the semantic analysis with the use of structural analysis very effective and efficient.

Of course, one can also point to some disadvantages of this approach, too. Among them the major one is frequent lack of an explicitly set grammar for a given task and a need to construct it on the basis of a vast test data set or even based on the developed features vector. The structure of the correct grammar requires that a series of inferences be drawn in order to determine the optimal set of derivation rules, which will form a grammar generating the looked-for language. This task, however, is not always easy due to that, for example, there is no uniqueness between the languages given and grammars formulated for them (frequently they generate a more extensive language).

The wish to develop a compact grammar notation for a given task can encounter also other difficulties associated with the use of one of grammar classes for which it is difficult to develop (automatically) software translators of the analysed language expressions. Within the group of sequential grammars, the 0-type grammars (phrase-structure grammars) have the greatest derivation capacity and it is them that enable the development of the shortest grammar derivations possible. Unfortunately, the easier a grammar is formulated, the more difficult it is to execute the parsing tasks. When the formalisms are too strong, it is not possible to use effectively the available programming tools for creation of automatic translation modules. In practical applications, context-free grammars prove to be the most effective class since with them one can literally chose from among ready-made grammar compilers.

As far as the analysis of images considered in this book is concerned, the technique of understanding the image semantics is characterised by a number of advantages.

The main advantage of context-free grammar use, as compared to methods of analysis developed by other researchers is that it allows for the diagnosing of both concentric changes (e.g. *stenoses*) seen on a cross-section as a uniform stricture of the whole lumen as well as eccentric changes (e.g. *stenoses*) occurring only on one organ or vessel wall. This fact is important from the point of view of diagnosis since it helps us recognise whether the discovered symptom is characteristic for a specified lesion e.g. stable disturbance of heart rhythm (in the case of diagnosed concentric stricture) or for unstable angina (when an eccentric *stenosis* is discovered).

The thresholds of a few percent of the misidentified lesions in the test data sets in each case result from the non-optimal selection of the approximation accuracy thresholds of the width diagram for particular kind of images. In the research conducted, this size has been defined as 2 pixels for all cases, with image resolution of 300 dpi. Due to the fact, however, that the width profile approximation procedure can determine the value of the approximation threshold in a dynamic manner, an increase in the recognition efficiency requires that its value be dependent on the size of the analysed vessel or organ lumen. In the case of smaller lumen the approximation threshold should be respectively smaller. That will result in making it sensitive to small and subtle changes. In the case of bigger organs the threshold can be relatively bigger since as a result of approximation the individual contour points do not lose important diagnostic information determined by semantic actions. This solution shall be considered in further research aimed at improvement of the presented technique of image understanding and of the performance and standardisation of the method involving an analysis of a much larger set of data of medical images.

The research undertaken so far reveals that the approach proposed in this paper can be an extremely efficient and universal tool enabling visual data compression and unambiguous data representation. An important point is that the proposed perception technique is optimised and targeted at diagnostic information observable in the shape of organs visible on patterns and dependent on disease symptoms present there.

The main strength of the proposed structural methods for understanding data in medical visual data bases is its high efficiency resulting from small memory complexity of semantic representation generated to represent patterns. This approach is also insensitive to minor disturbances (noise) or geometrical transformations of patterns since these factors are independent of the generated syntactic and semantic representation.

In the examples of coronography, urographic patterns and pancreas visualisation presented in the study, a semantic descriptor created with the use of the described methodology allows us to diagnose a concrete disease on the basis of a single pattern; it serves also as a key for indexation in searching for data in the data base. Those properties result from the unambiguity of representation generated for various semantic contents.

In practical terms the result of computer implementation of the syntactic analysis algorithms provided in this study is the development of a system allowing for structural analysis of the discussed medical patterns with a view to creating a semantic representation defining various disease symptoms. The research confirmed that there is potential for developing an adequate description for visible deformations of shapes as well as for the semantic categorisation of various disease symptoms. Those descriptions can be used as results of important lesions recognition. Yet, from the point of view of knowledge engineering, they may constitute also a data set for deeper reasoning and may be used in Computer-Aided Diagnosis.

References

1. Bellon EM (1983) Radiologic Interpretation of ERCP: a Clinical Atlas. Medical Examination Publishing Co., New York
2. Berchtold S, Keim DA, Kriegel HP, Seidl T (2000) Indexing the solution space: a new technique for nearest neighbor search in high-dimensional space. IEEE Transactions on Knowledge & Data Engineering 12(1):45–57
3. Bertrand G, Everat J-Ch, Couprie M (1997) Image segmentation through operators based on topology. Journal of Electronic Imaging 6(4):395–405
4. Bunke H, Haller B (1990) A parser for context free plex grammars, LNCS 411:136–402
5. Duda RO, Hart PE, Stork DG (2001) Pattern classifications (2nd ed.). Willey
6. Flasiński M (1993) On the parsing of deterministic graph languages for syntactic pattern recognition. Pattern Recognition 26:1–16
7. Gao Q (1998) Man-made object recognition based on visual perception. Journal of Electronic Imaging 7(1):104–110
8. Hall P, Ngan M, Andreae P (1998) Reconstructing vascular skeletons from X-ray angiograms. In: Hanson KM (eds) Medical Imaging 1998: Image Processing, Proceedings of SPIE Vol. 3338, pp 480–491
9. Hasenplaugh WC, Neifeld MA (1999) Image binarization techniques for correlation-based pattern recognition. Optical Engineering 38(11):1907–1917
10. Khan MG (1996) Heart Disease Diagnosis and Therapy. Williams & Wilkins, Baltimore
11. Kurgan LA, Cios KJ, Tadeusiewicz R, Ogiela MR, Goodenday LS (2001) Knowledge Discovery Approach to Automated Cardiac SPECT Diagnosis. Artificial Intelligence in Medicine 23(2):149–189
12. Leondes CT (eds) (1998) Image processing and pattern recognition. Academic Press, San Diego
13. Leś Z, Tadeusiewicz R (2000) Shape Understanding System - Generating Exemplars Of The Polygon Class. In: Hamza MH, Sarfraz E (eds.) Computer Graphics and Imaging. IASTED/ACTA Press, Anaheim, Calgary, Zurich, pp 139–144
14. Leś Z, Tadeusiewicz R (2000) Shape Understanding System, Polygon Class Processing Methods. in Hamza MH (eds) Signal Processing and Communications. IASTED/ACTA Press, Anaheim, Calgary, Zurich, pp 447–454
15. Leś Z, Tadeusiewicz R, Leś M (2001) Shape Understanding: Knowledge Generation and Learning. In: Proceedings of the Seventh Australian and New Zealand Intelligent Information Systems Conference (ANZIIS 2001), IEEE

Engineering in Medicine and Biology Society, Perth, Western Australia, pp 189–195
16. Levine J, Mason T, Brown D (1992) LEX & YACC. O'Reilly & Associates, Inc.
17. Mancini GB (eds) (1988) Clinical Applications of Cardiac Digital Angiography. Raven Press, New York
18. Mandal AK, Jennette JCh (eds.) (1994) Diagnosis and Management of Renal Disease and Hypertension. Carolina Academic Press
19. Martinez AM, Serra JR (2000) A new approach to object-related image retrieval. Journal of Visual Languages & Computing 11(3):345–363
20. Miclet L (1986) Structural methods in pattern recognition. Springer-Verlag
21. Mikrut Z (1996) A Method of Linear Star-Sections Applied for Object Separation in ERCP Images. In: Proceedings of International Conference on Image Processing, Lausanne, pp. 363–366
22. Netter FH, Colacino S (1998) Atlas of Human Anatomy. Novartis Medical Education
23. Niu Y, Mtamer Ozsu, Xiaobo Li (1999) 2-D-S tree: An index structure for content-based retrieval of images. In: Proceedings of SPIE Vol. 3654, pp 110–121
24. Ogiela MR (1998) Languages of shape feature description and syntactic methods for recognition of morphological changes of organs in analysis of selected X-ray images. In: Hanson KM (eds) Medical Imaging 1998: Image Processing, Proceedings of SPIE Vol. 3338, pp 1295–1305
25. Ogiela, MR, Tadeusiewicz R (1997) Recognition of some types X-ray images for medical diagnosis. Biocybernetics and Biomedical Engineering 17(3–4):69–91
26. Ogiela MR, Tadeusiewicz R (1998) Computer Recognition of X-ray Images for Medical Diagnosis. In: Togawa T, Nałęcz M (eds) Lecture Notes of the ICB Seminars; 2nd Japan-Polish Seminar on Contribution of Electrical and Electronic Engineering to Biology and Medicine, pp 263–282
27. Ogiela MR, Tadeusiewicz R (1999) Syntactic Analysis and Languages of Shape Feature Description in Computer Aided Diagnosis and Recognition of Cancerous and Inflammatory Lesions of Organs in Selected X-Ray Images. Journal of Digital Imaging 12(2) Suppl 1:24–27
28. Ogiela MR, Tadeusiewicz R (1999) Application of Selected Artificial Intelligence Methods for Medical X-Ray Images. In: Piecha J. (eds) Medical Information Technology (TIM'99), Jaszowiec 1999, pp 1–14
29. Ogiela MR, Tadeusiewicz R (2000) Artificial Intelligence Methods in Shape Feature Analysis of Selected Organs in Medical Images. Image Processing & Communications 6(1–2):3–11
30. Ogiela MR, Tadeusiewicz R (2000) Syntactic pattern recognition for X-ray diagnosis of pancreatic cancer. IEEE Engineering In Medicine and Biology Magazine 19(6):94–105
31. Ogiela MR, Tadeusiewicz R (2000) Syntactic Methods of Shape Feature Description and Its Application in Analysis of Medical Images. In: Erbacher RF,

Chen PC, Roberts JC, Wittenbrink CM (eds) Visual Data Exploration and Analysis VII, Proceedings of SPIE Vol. 3960, pp 326–333

32. Ogiela MR, Tadeusiewicz R (2000) Application of Syntactic Methods of Pattern Recognition for Data Mining and Knowledge Discovery in Medicine. In: Dasarathy BV (eds), Data Mining and Knowledge Discovery: Theory, Tool, and Technology II, , Proceedings of SPIE Vol. 4057, pp 308–318
33. Ogiela MR, Tadeusiewicz R (2000) Mathematical linguistics methods and their application for recognition of pathological signs in medical images. In: Proceedings of the NORSIG 2000 – IEEE Nordic Signal Processing Symposium, Kolmarden, Sweden, pp 267–270
34. Ogiela MR, Tadeusiewicz R (2001) Image Understanding Methods in Biomedical Informatics and Digital Imaging. Journal of Biomedical Informatics 34(6):377–386
35. Ogiela MR, Tadeusiewicz R (2001) Advances in syntactic imaging techniques for perception of medical images. The Imaging Science Journal 49(2):113–120
36. Ogiela MR, Tadeusiewicz R (2001) Automatic understanding of selected diseases on the base of structural analysis of medical images. In: Proceedings of the 2001 IEEE International Conference on Acoustics, Speech, and Signal Processing (ICASSP 2001), Salt Lake City, Utah, USA, Vol. III, pp 2009–2012
37. Ogiela MR, Tadeusiewicz R (2001) Semantic-Oriented Syntactic Algorithms for Content Recognition and Understanding of Images in Medical Data bases. In: Proceedings of the 2001 IEEE International Conference on Multimedia and Expo- ICME 2001, Tokyo, Japan, pp 621–624
38. Ogiela MR, Tadeusiewicz R (2001) Intelligent Information Systems for Visual Data Understanding and Analysis. In: Engemann KJ, Lasker GE (eds) Proceedings of the 13th International Conference on Systems Research, Informatics and Cybernetics (INTERSYMP-2001), Baden-Baden, Germany, Advances in Decision technology and Intelligent Information Systems, Vol 2, pp 18–22
39. Ogiela MR, Tadeusiewicz R (2001) New Aspects of Using the Structural Graph-Grammar Based Techniques for Recognition of Selected Medical Images. Journal of Digital Imaging 14(2) Suppl 1:231–232
40. Ogiela MR, Tadeusiewicz R (2002) Syntactic reasoning and pattern recognition for analysis of coronary artery images. Artificial Intelligence in Medicine 26:145–159
41. Ogiela MR, Tadeusiewicz R (2002) Advanced image understanding and pattern analysis methods in Medical Imaging. In: *Proceedings of the Fourth IASTED International Conference SIGNAL and IMAGE PROCESSING (SIP 2002)*, Kaua'i, Hawaii, USA, pp 583–588
42. Ogiela MR, Tadeusiewicz R (2003) Visual Signal Processing and Image Understanding in Biomedical Systems. In: Proceedings of the 2003 IEEE International Symposium on Circuits and Systems, Vol. 5, Bangkok 2003, pp V-17 – V-20

43. Ogiela MR, Tadeusiewicz R (2003) Artificial Intelligence Structural Imaging Techniques in Visual Pattern Analysis and Medical Data Understanding. Pattern Recognition 36(10):2441–2452
44. Ogiela MR, Tadeusiewicz R (2003) Nonlinear Processing and Semantic Content Analysis in Medical Imaging. In: Processing of IEEE International Symposium on Intelligent Signal Processing entitled 'From classical measurement to computing with perceptions', Budapest WISP 2003, pp 243–247
45. Ogiela MR, Tadeusiewicz R, Ogiela L (2002) Syntactic Pattern Analysis in Visual Signal Processing and Image Understanding. In: Proceedings of The International Conference on Fundamentals of Electronic, Communications and Computer Science – ICFS 2002, Tokyo, Japan, pp 13:10 – 13:14
46. Ogiela MR, Tadeusiewicz R, Ogiela L (2002) Development of Intelligent Medical Pattern Perception Systems. In: Proceedings D of the 5th International Multi-Conference, Information Society - IS'2002, Development and Reengineering of Information Systems, Ljubljana Slovenia, pp 251–254
47. Ogiela MR, Tadeusiewicz R, Ogiela L (2002) Intelligent Image Understanding Systems. In: Proceedings A of the 5th International Multi-Conference, Information Society - IS'2002, Intelligent Systems, Ljubljana Slovenia, pp 35–38
48. Ogiela MR, Tadeusiewicz R, Ogiela L (2003) Content-based Reasoning in Intelligent Medical Information System. In: Proceedings of ICEIS 2003: Fifth International Conference on Enterprise Information Systems, ESEO-AAAI-ACM-ASTI-IEEE Computer Society, Angers (France), pp 503–506
49. Pavlidis T (1982) Algorithms for Graphics and Image Processing. Computer Science Press, Rockville
50. Siegel EL, Reiner BI (1999) Challenges associated with incorporation of digital radiography into a Picture Archiving and Communications System. Journal of Digital Imaging 12(2) Suppl. 1:6–8
51. Silvus SE, Rohrmann ChA, Ansel HJ (1995) Text and atlas of endoscopic retrograde cholangiopancreatography. Igaku-Shain, New York
52. Singh S, Haddon J, Markou M (1999) Nearest neighbour strategies for image understanding. In: Blanc-Talon J, Popescu D (eds) The International Institute for Advanced Studies in Systems Research and Cybernetics, pp 74–79
53. Sklansky J, Gonzales V (1980) Fast Polygonal Approximation of Digitized Curves. Pattern Recognition 12:327–331
54. Skomorowski M (1998) Use of random graphs for scene analysis. Machine Graphics & Vision 7:313–323
55. Sonka M, Fitzpatrick JM (eds) (2000) Handbook of Medical Imaging: Vol. 2- Medical Image Processing and Analysis. SPIE PRESS Vol. PM80
56. Tadeusiewicz R, Flasinski M (1991) Pattern recognition (in Polish). Polish Scientific Publisher, Warsaw
57. Tadeusiewicz R, Ogiela MR (2001) Structural Methods for X-Ray Pattern recognition. In: Heeren G. (eds): Teaching Course on Imaging for Target Volume Determination in Radiotherapy (ESTRO 2001), European Society for Therapeutic Radiology and Oncology, ESTRO Krakow, pp1 – 10

58. Tadeusiewicz R, Ogiela MR (2001) Automatic Understanding of Medical Images, New Achievements in Syntactic Analysis of Selected Medical Images. In: 5th Polish-Japanese Seminar on Biomedical Measurements. New Methods for Medical Diagnosis, Zakopane p 32
59. Tadeusiewicz R, Ogiela MR (2001) Examples of the Application of New Approach to Structural Analysis of Medical Images. Archive of Theoretical and Applied Computer Science 13(4):311–327
60. Tadeusiewicz R, Ogiela MR (2001) Automatic Understanding of Medical Images. New achievements in Syntactic Analysis of Selected Medical Images; In: Togawa T, Nałęcz M (eds) Lecture Notes of the ICB Seminars; 5th Japan-Polish Seminar on Biomedical Measurements – New Methods for Medical Diagnosis, International Center of Biocybernetics, 56: 84–94
61. Tadeusiewicz R, Ogiela MR (2002) Automatic Understanding Of Medical Images - New Achievements In Syntactic Analysis Of Selected Medical Images. Biocybernetics and Biomedical Engineering 22(4):17–29
62. Tadeusiewicz R, Ogiela MR (2003) Artificial Intelligence Techniques in Retrieval of Visual Data Semantic Information. In: Menasalvas E, Segovia J, Szczepaniak PS (eds) Advances in Web Intelligence, LNAI 2663, Springer Verlag, pp 18–27
63. Tadeusiewicz R, Ogiela MR (2003) Machine Perception and Automatic Understanding of Medical Visualisations. In: Damczyk M. (eds) Automatic Image Processing in Production Process, Second Polish-German Seminar, CAMT, Wroclaw 2003, pp 39–48
64. Tanaka E (1995) Theoretical aspects of syntactic pattern recognition. Pattern Recognition 28:1053–1061
65. Waite WM, Goos G (1984) Compiler Construction.Springer-Verlag, New York
66. Wszołek W, Tadeusiewicz R, Izworski A, Wszołek T (2002) Recognition and Understanding of The Pathological Speech Using Artificial Intelligence Methods. In: Hamza MH (eds) Artificial Intelligence and Applications, IASTED, ACTA Press Anaheim-Calgary-Zurich, pp 504–508

Index

Printing: Strauss GmbH, Mörlenbach
Binding: Schäffer, Grünstadt